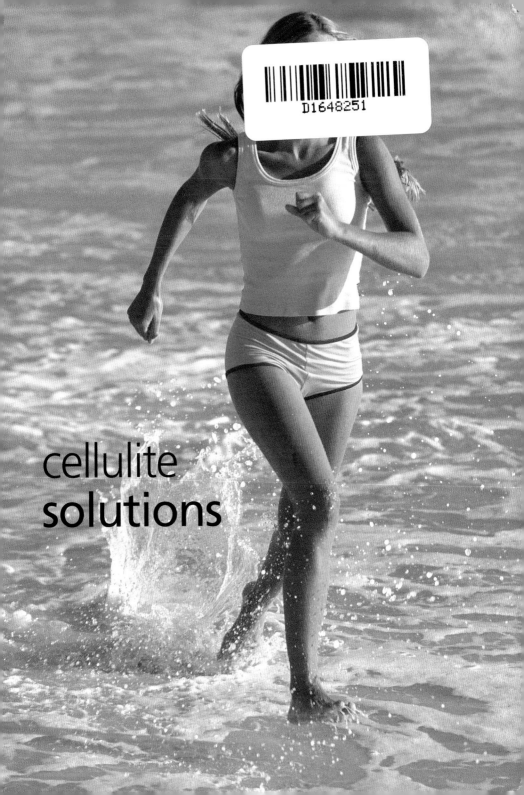

cellulite
solutions

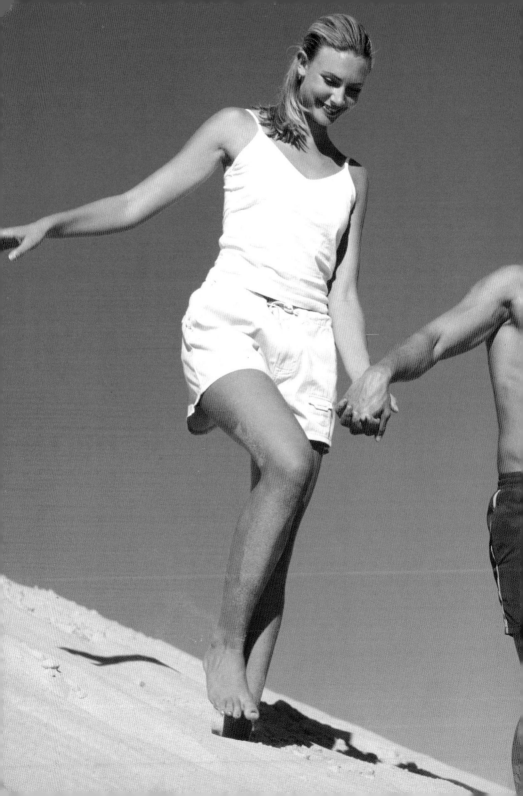

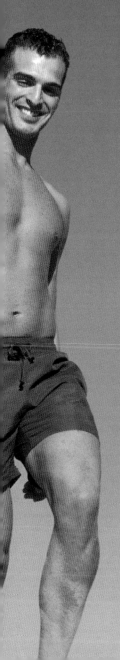

hamlyn

cellulite
solutions

7 ways to beat cellulite in 6 weeks

helen foster

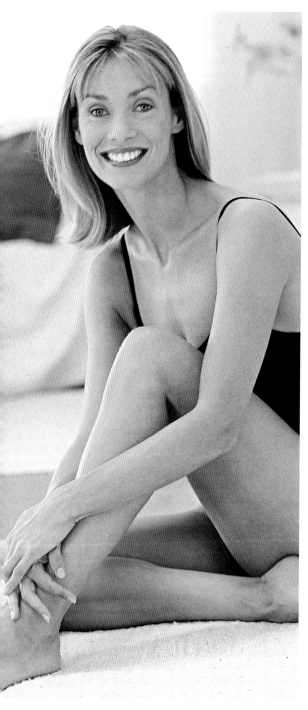

A Pyramid Paperback from Hamlyn

First published in Great Britain in 2003 by
Hamlyn, a division of
Octopus Publishing Group Ltd
2–4 Heron Quays, London E14 4JP

This material was previously published as
Cellulite Solutions. This revised edition
published 2007

Distributed in the United States and
Canada by
Sterling Publishing Co., Inc.
387 Park Avenue South,
New York, NY 10016-8810

ISBN 10 0 600 61605 3
ISBN 13 978 0 600 61605 4

A CIP catalogue record for this book is
available from the British Library

Printed in China

10 9 8 7 6 5 4 3 2 1

Safety note
This book should not be considered a
replacement for professional medical
treatment; a physician should be consulted
on all matters relating to health. While the
advice and information in this book is
believed to be accurate, neither the author
nor publisher can accept any legal
responsibility for any injury or illness
sustained while following it.

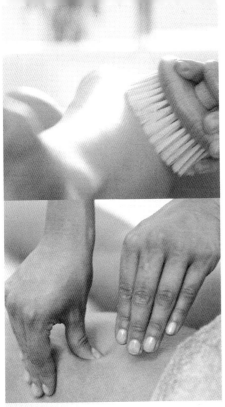

contents

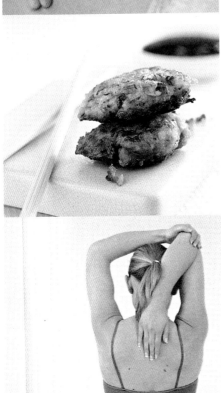

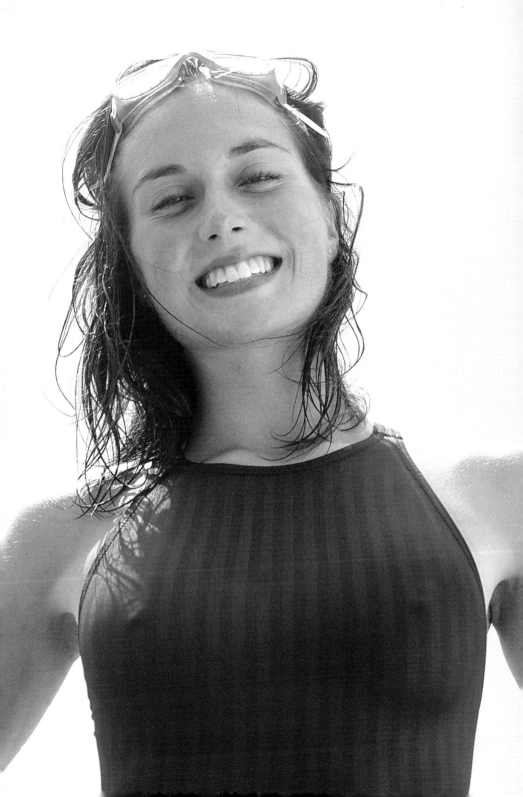

introduction

Cosmetic experts have estimated that 90 per cent of women in the western world have some kind of cellulite. They can be tall women, small women, thin women or fat women – even supermodels and actresses who are paid millions to keep themselves in shape can't escape it.

You probably don't remember exactly when you first spotted it. You may have been standing in front of the mirror when the light from behind you revealed grey shadows and less than smooth skin. Or maybe you first noticed it when you crossed your legs and suddenly, as the skin was squashed, grey bumps and white lumps appeared. Whenever you first noticed you had cellulite, there was probably one thought that raced through your mind: how do I get rid of it? Once cellulite appears, nearly all women want it gone.

The good news is that there has never been a better time to tackle cellulite, because science has finally caught up. When I started writing about health and fitness back in the 1980s, doctors denied its existence. Now doctors, cosmetic surgeons and scientists not only believe that cellulite exists, but they are looking into exactly what it is and how to fight it.

The result is that never before has so much information been collected about cellulite. Rather than just saying it's something women have to put up with, scientists are now putting cellulite under the microscope and finding out exactly what makes this lumpy, bumpy fat different from the fat elsewhere on our bodies. The more they know about it, the more it allows them to come up with ways to fight cellulite. Nutritional approaches, supplements, creams and alternative therapies are all being investigated as beauty companies and the medical profession race to be the first to find that one thing that will banish those bumps forever.

Unfortunately I'm not going to be the person to reveal the miracle cure: as yet, no one has found it. However, I can outline a whole host of little things which, when put together in a simple regime, can help fight cellulite. This book combines traditional therapies for cellulite with the latest research trials, revealing new and exciting ways to combat it. You will be taught the ultimate cellulite-fighting plan that will reduce – or even remove – your cellulite within just six weeks.

But that's not the only benefit to be had from this programme. Because it helps fight weight gain and fluid retention, after following the plan your whole body is going to end up slimmer and firmer – not just your hips and thighs. Because the plan relies on high-nutrient foods, your body will never have felt or looked healthier, your energy levels will improve, your hair and skin are likely to get a beauty boost and you could even find you get ill less often. By following the exercises you will boost your strength and stamina and lower your risk of problems like heart disease and cancer.

Finally, by using a whole host of techniques to fight the free radicals that cause ageing (and contribute to cellulite) you can help your body feel and look younger. In fact, the techniques you will be using over the next six weeks won't just transform the way you feel about your cellulite, but your whole body. Think of it as a total overhaul that has the added benefit of making you look better in a swimsuit. But before we start the overhaul, it is important to get back to basics and focus on exactly what cellulite really is.

what is cellulite?

Cellulite is generally defined as dimpled skin that appears, most commonly, on the hips and thighs. At first it appears only when the skin is pressed (for example, when you cross your legs), but as it develops it is visible all the time and creates dips and dimples on the skin's surface.

Cellulite can feel strange to the touch. Some women say it is hard, cold and actually quite painful when it's pressed or massaged. Others report it as spongy and doughy. Many women have patches of both types of cellulite. However, looks aren't everything and what truly determines the nature of cellulite is not what you see on the surface of the skin, but what is happening underneath. And until recently, nobody really knew what cellulite was.

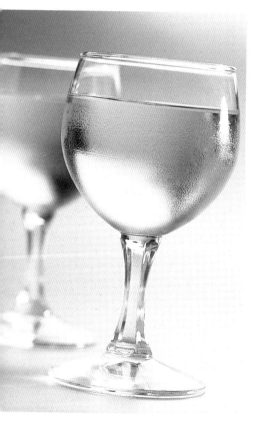

Despite the fact that there had been references in scientific literature for 150 years about this strange dimply fat that affected women's hips and thighs, until about 1998 nobody had ever studied it properly. The popular theory was that cellulite was caused by toxins from alcohol, caffeine, nicotine and red meat, and that these toxins, unable to be processed by the body, were pushed into the fat stores. As these stores got fuller and fuller, the toxins began to bulge out against the skin, creating doming and dimpling.

There is a scientific basis for this theory as the body does push toxins that it can't handle into the fat stores. However, it is not the little toxins like caffeine or red meat that it processes in this way, it is big toxins such as heavy metals found in air pollution or pesticides on foods.

This was why those working in the medical profession didn't really believe the toxin theory – after all, if caffeine, alcohol and smoking were the cause of cellulite, why didn't more men get it? They are just as likely as women to drink coffee, smoke or drink alcohol night after night.

The answer was revealed in June 1998. A team from New York's Rockefeller University looked in detail at cellulite for the first time – and what they found changed everything. When they analysed samples of tissue affected by cellulite they didn't find traces of caffeine, red meat or nicotine. Similarly, they didn't find abnormally high traces of heavy metals or pesticides. Instead they found normal fat, the same as appears on your tummy and on other bits of your hips and thighs. However, what was different about this fat was the way it was held in place within the skin.

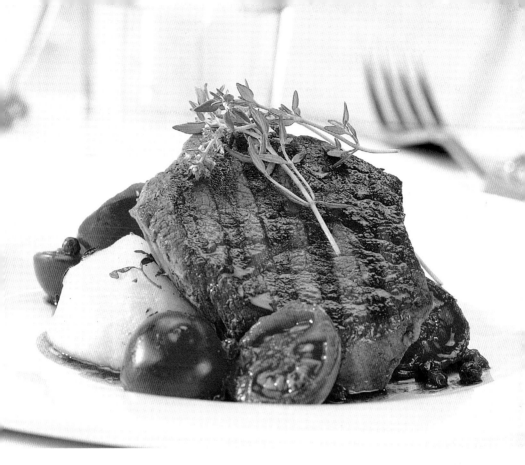

THE SKIN PROBLEM

All around our bodies, we have an important layer of fat under the skin called the subcutis. This is what keeps us warm, cushions us when we sit down and protects our bones. Through this fat layer run fibres of collagen (called septa) that collect the fat into pockets. These septa are attached to the underside of the skin and the outer part of the muscle underneath and they keep the fat in place.

The Rockefeller research team found that in men, these fibres run diagonally against the skin, pressing down on the fat and keeping it smooth. However, in women, the fibres run straight up and down, creating tall, thin rectangular boxes with nothing pushing them downwards. This means that if the fat cells within these 'boxes' get bigger or more numerous (both of which

IS CELLULITE HEREDITARY?

It could be. It's certainly true of facial ageing that what happens to your mother will happen to you – and facial ageing is primarily controlled by the strength of collagen and elastin. If they are weak in the face, they could also be weak elsewhere on the body. Finally, there can also be a genetic link to weight gain, which may make it easier for some people to gain weight; and the more fat you have, the more likely it is that you will have cellulite.

occur when you gain weight), nothing would stop the excess volume bulging out over the top of the 'box', creating a domed look.

What this didn't explain was why it affected thin women too – after all they don't have excess fat to bulge out. Further research then found two more differences in the cellulite areas. The first is that in cellulite, the septa actually differ in structure from those in normal fat. Instead of being thin strips of collagen, they are thicker and press sideways on the fat, squashing it upwards and increasing the bulging and doming effect even where fat stores are limited.

The second difference was found by a research team at the University of Florence in Italy. They discovered that cellulite actually contains higher than average levels of water-attracting cells called proteoglycans. This means that any fluid entering areas of cellulite is more likely to be retained there, and this too could bulge up underneath the skin.

So the next question is why does this happen? What turns normal fat-filled areas into patches

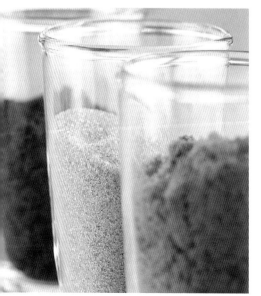

of cellulite? As yet nobody really knows, but it's increasingly looking as if two factors are involved – free-radical attack and poor circulation. They could work together, they could work alone, but they do seem to explain the problem.

FREE RADICALS

Free radicals are compounds that are created in our bodies when we are exposed to toxins from smoking, alcohol, air pollution, pesticides and even some relatively harmless food ingredients such as fats and sugars. The problem with free radicals is that they are missing an electron and to make themselves complete they have to steal an electron from a cell somewhere in the body. As they do this, they start to attack and degrade those cells.

While free-radical damage can happen to any cell in the body, the compounds seem to have a particular affinity for collagen and elastin cells that make up the top layers of the skin and this can have a number of effects on cellulite. When collagen and elastin degrade, the skin thins. This reduces the covering over the subcutis, making any overfilled fat 'boxes' a lot more noticeable.

Also, as the septa are actually made up of collagen, free radicals will attack them directly. This makes the septa tougher and less elastic, causing them to shorten and pull down on the skin's surface. To make matters worse, when the body tries to repair the damage, the second potential trigger for cellulite comes into play.

IS CELLULITE HARMFUL?
Cellulite is not an illness, nor has it been linked to any medical conditions. Other than perhaps making you feel unhappy, cellulite itself will not have any ill effects on your health. However, it may be a sign that your lifestyle isn't as healthy as it could be – and this may affect your general health.

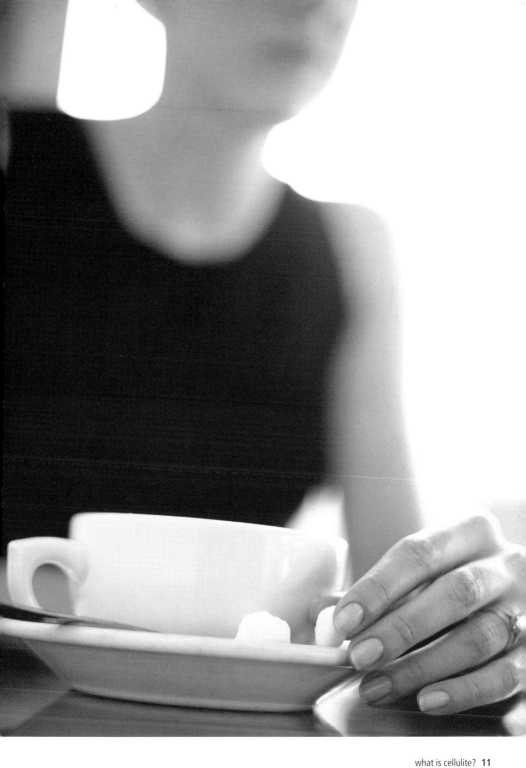

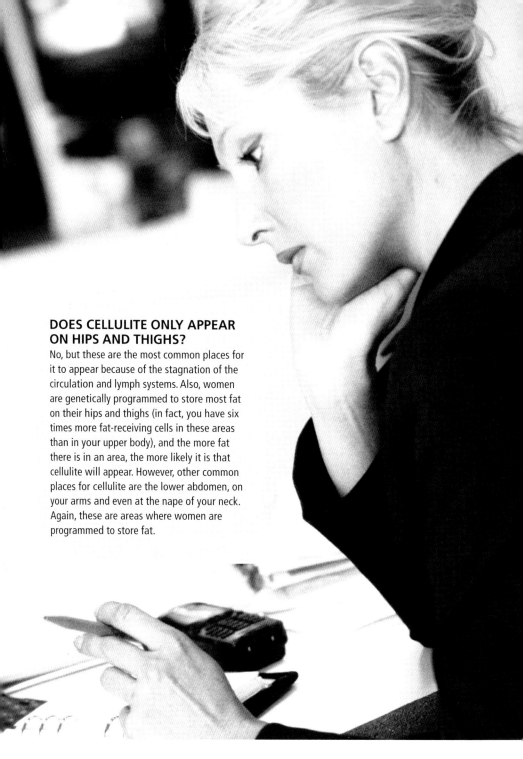

DOES CELLULITE ONLY APPEAR ON HIPS AND THIGHS?

No, but these are the most common places for it to appear because of the stagnation of the circulation and lymph systems. Also, women are genetically programmed to store most fat on their hips and thighs (in fact, you have six times more fat-receiving cells in these areas than in your upper body), and the more fat there is in an area, the more likely it is that cellulite will appear. However, other common places for cellulite are the lower abdomen, on your arms and even at the nape of your neck. Again, these are areas where women are programmed to store fat.

BAD CIRCULATION

This second trigger is sluggish circulation and a poorly performing lymphatic system. According to research carried out by Dr Sergio Curri at the Centre of Molecular Biology in Milan, and a further study at Brussels University, areas of cellulite suffer from both of these problems. The job of the circulatory system in the body is to carry oxygen and nutrients to all cells, while the lymphatic system carries away toxic by-products.

Both systems are often stagnated in our hips and thighs. In these regions, both systems have to flow upwards, which is hard work at the best of times. Add to this the fact that many of us have sedentary jobs, which mean the hips and thighs are squashed into chairs all day and on the sofa all night. There are also the fashion foibles that many of us live with that mean we spend all day squashed into tight jeans, nipped-in waistbands or even control-top underwear. It is easy to see that the circulation and lymph systems have a difficult job.

And this can compound the cellulite problem. When they are deprived of oxygen (as they are if circulation slows), cells in the skin called fibroblasts (which normally create healthy tissue) start to clump together. When they are called on to repair the damaged collagen in the septa, instead of creating thin, healthy fibres they create thick, stringy fibres.

If lymph circulation is poor, the lymph fluid also solidifies and creates thickened fibres of its own that bind with the septa beneath the skin. These two processes in turn create thick strands that push harder on to the fat, making it bulge even further upwards.

What's more, poor circulation and lymph flow also result in fluids staying in the area longer than normal. As explained earlier, the higher levels of water-attracting cells within cellulite mean that it acts rather like a sponge and collects excess fluid.

Put simply, cellulite is a mix of fat cells swollen by fluid, being pressed on by thick, hard fibres that cause those fat cells to bulge out from the skin like the stuffing in an old sofa. And to beat cellulite, it is this combination of factors you have to tackle. But before we get to the solution, we need to understand why the body breaks down in the first place, so let's look at the causes of cellulite.

WHY DO SOME PEOPLE HAVE MORE CELLULITE THAN OTHERS?

Cellulite develops in stages, so what you see is determined by which stage you are at. How easy your cellulite will be to fight is also determined by how far it is developed. It is therefore good to know how severe yours is, so you can be more realistic about what you're going to achieve over the next six weeks. While severe cellulite will reduce in six weeks, it will take longer to get rid of it completely. Minor cellulite may disappear completely in even less than the six weeks recommended. These are the stages:

minor You can only see the cellulite if you pinch it with your fingers.

mild You can only see the cellulite if you are sitting down.

moderate Cellulite shows through the skin when you are standing up, but is mainly concentrated on the backs of the hips, bottom and thighs.

severe This appears when you are standing, in areas other than the back of your hips, bottom and thighs – and is taut or painful when you squash it.

the causes of cellulite

So far we have discussed what is happening under the skin when cellulite forms, but it is also important to understand what triggers this process. After six weeks on the cellulite-busting plan, you will need to avoid these triggers or the cellulite will reappear.

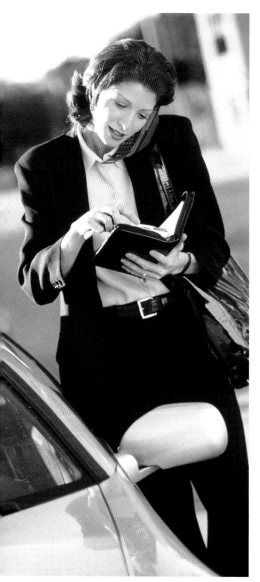

This section looks at some of the potential causes of cellulite and examines why they may make it form. While scientists have made progress determining what cellulite is, they haven't yet discovered exactly why it appears. The following are the most likely suspects.

AGE

While cellulite can start to appear at any time after puberty, it becomes more common after the age of 30. There are several reasons for this. To start with, from the age of 30, the average woman gains 4.5–6.8 kg (10–15 lb) of fat per decade, and the more fat you have on your body, the higher your risk of cellulite becomes. Ageing also triggers the thinning of the top layer of the skin that covers the subcutis layer, making the bumpy fat more visible from the surface. Finally, over the years collagen fibres start to harden. This means the septa, which tether the skin to the underlying muscle, start to shorten and the skin is pulled downwards – the cause of the dimpling you see on the surface.

SEDENTARY LIFESTYLES

Today we walk an average of 13 km (8 miles) per day less than our grandparents did – and every element of the formation of cellulite is affected by that inactivity. For example, the less you move, the fewer calories you will burn off and the more likely it is that you will gain weight. Inactivity also slows the circulation – when we exercise we strengthen the heart and without that strengthening, circulation is likely to be slowed. The problem is even worse for the lymph. It has no pump to send it round the system. Instead it relies solely on the contraction of the muscles and if you don't move regularly, the lymph flow will slow down.

EXCESS WEIGHT

In the UK, over 30 per cent of women are overweight, while 20 per cent are classed as obese. In the US, 35 per cent of the population is deemed overweight while a further 25 per cent are obese. This picture is echoed over much of the western world. While it's true that cellulite does affect slim women, cellulite is fat and overweight people are more prone to it.

SMOKING

While nobody has yet done conclusive research, it seems likely that smoking is a major contributing factor to cellulite. Smoking causes mass formation of free radicals, with millions entering the body with every puff. Also, researchers in Japan have found that smoking triggers the production of enzymes in the body called MMP (matrix metalloproteins). These chop up collagen fibres, causing skin to thin – and when this happens cellulite becomes more noticeable. And should your body try to repair that collagen, it's going to find it harder to do so, as smoking reduces the body's levels of vitamin C, the nutrient that is essential for the formation of collagen.

OTHER TOXINS

There are a few other very common habits that may also contribute to cellulite, namely drinking too much alcohol, relying on caffeine and eating too many fatty or sugary foods. While it may not be correct to say that these things cause cellulite by clogging up the fat cells with their debris, it doesn't mean they're not involved in its formation. For starters, all of the above create free radicals and trigger stress on the lymph system. They also destroy some of the vital nutrients we need to actually burn fat off. For example, each cup of coffee knocks 6mg of calcium from your stores – and calcium helps convert cells from fat-storers to fat-burners.

SUNBATHING

One of the nastiest factors in the fight against cellulite is that tanning – one of the few things that disguises the dimples – could actually be contributing to your problem. In high summer it takes as little as four minutes of sun exposure for damage to start occurring to the collagen and elastin fibres under the skin. And just like the effects of ageing or smoking, this damage thins the skin over the subcutis and makes cellulite much more noticeable. As well as this, exposure to too much sunlight dehydrates the skin and cellulite is also more noticeable on very dehydrated skin, as this causes it to become thinner and less flexible.

ARE YOU OVERWEIGHT?

To find out if you are overweight, you need to measure your body mass index (BMI). To do this, follow this simple formula:

$$BMI = \frac{\text{weight (kg)}}{\text{height (m) x height (m)}}$$

If the figure is between 25 and 29.9: you are carrying some excess weight and reducing this may help your cellulite (and your overall health).

If the figure is over 30: you are severely overweight and really should start to slim down, for all health reasons.

Note: If you are extremely athletic and have a very high muscle mass, it will skew the measurements. Ask your trainer or someone at your gym to do a body fat measurement and advise you accordingly.

DEHYDRATION

A recent paper in the *Journal of the American Dietetic Association* estimated that at any one time, up to 27 per cent of us are suffering from dehydration. Dehydration causes us to think more slowly, makes us more prone to headaches and mood swings, and causes our bodies to retain as much water as possible. One of the most common causes of fluid retention – and the cellulite that this can trigger – is dehydration. You need to drink plenty of liquid for your body to release the water it is storing. The good news is this doesn't have to be just water – weak tea, orange juice, tonic water, milk and decaffeinated diet drinks all supply fluid. Aim for the equivalent of eight glasses of fluid a day.

FOOD INTOLERANCES

These occur when the body loses the ability to digest certain types of food properly. This means the food hangs around the system longer than it should do and ferments, filling the body with toxic substances. The body reacts by trying to dilute the toxins with water, which can collect in the cellulite. The most common dietary intolerances are for wheat or dairy products. The symptoms are headaches, bloating, cramping or lethargy after eating the problem food – the symptoms vanish if you don't eat them for a few days. You may also gain more than 1.4–2.2 kg (3–4 lb) of weight in a day if you eat a lot of the problem food – caused by water retention as the body tries to dilute the toxins. If you think you are intolerant to dairy products, switch to calcium-fortified soya milk or orange juice instead of milk on your cereal to boost your calcium intake, and cut out cheese and yogurt.

HORMONES

It has often been suggested that exposure to the female hormone oestrogen can be a trigger for cellulite. There's a whole host of reasons for this: cellulite isn't normally triggered until puberty when oestrogen kicks in; it may get worse during pregnancy and the menopause when oestrogen levels go slightly haywire; and oestrogen has a tendency to encourage fluid retention and fat storage. However, there's another school of thought that says it's not the presence of oestrogen that contributes to cellulite, but the absence of testosterone. Testosterone leads to firmer, stronger connective fibres under the skin, which reduces the risk of the fat 'poking through' the top layer of skin. Obviously it's not desirable to increase levels of testosterone in the female body, but you can reduce the amount of oestrogen by keeping your weight down, as fat tissue actually creates its own low levels of oestrogen.

STRESS

Studies have shown that it is possible that stress may contribute to cellulite. When you are stressed the muscles in your body tense, particularly in the back and neck. This blocks the flow of lymph. In addition to this, stress is also a major cause of weight gain. Not only does it make you comfort-eat, but stress also increases levels of a hormone called cortisol and this is a major appetite stimulator. Cortisol also makes the abdominal cells more prone to collecting fat. If you carry a proportionately large amount of excess weight around your middle or have cellulite on your stomach, stress is likely to be a major factor.

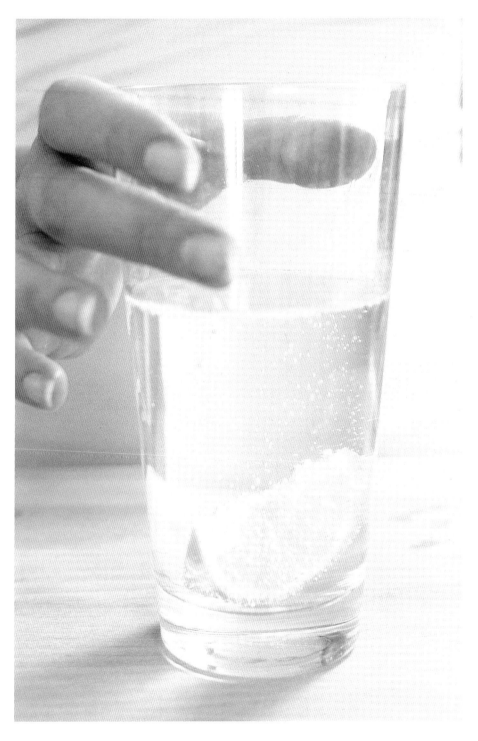

how the solutions work

By discovering the potential triggers for cellulite it may seem that our lifestyles are geared towards it. Exercise is a good example. It can make a big difference to cellulite, yet 70 per cent of people in the UK don't exercise more than once a month – and only 40 per cent of Americans do.

We are just as bad when it comes to what we eat: two of the major food factors believed to trigger cellulite are sugar and fat. The average British diet contains roughly 9 kg (20 lb) of sugar a year and 35 kg (77 lb) of fat, both too high for good health. The average American consumes about 10 per cent less fat, but three times as much sugar. The truth is that for most of us, cellulite is virtually unavoidable – but all that is about to change for you.

The Solutions that follow can actually tackle all the physiological causes of cellulite. This book offers seven different plans containing techniques that will help reduce – or even remove – your cellulite. For maximum benefit, follow all these Solutions together for the next six weeks. You will be using a multitude of techniques to reduce excess fat and fluid, rapidly decreasing the amount of cellulite you have. You will also start to reduce the amount of free radicals in your system and initiate repair of the damaged collagen under the skin, cutting down on the risk of it coming back.

It is best to read all the sections before you start because for optimum results they do need to be used at the same time. You may think there's a lot of information to remember, but simple at-a-glance guides in the longer sections tell you exactly what you should be doing when.

THE MIX-AND-MATCH APPROACH

If you are really pressed for time, it doesn't mean cellulite-free thighs are not for you. You will get some benefit simply by following the Diet and Exercise Solutions, and fitting in other Solutions as you can. If you are going to try this approach, add the other Solutions in the order that follows to really maximize results, while cutting down on the time you need to spend.

1 Take the supplements recommended in the Supplement Solution.

2 Apply a good cellulite cream (see page 106) or an aromatherapy blend (from the recommendations on page 95) nightly, using the manual lymph technique on page 88.

3 Spend five minutes skin brushing (see page 86) each morning.

4 Try to introduce the mental tips from the Psychological Solution into your daily thinking.

5 Use the other aromatherapy and hydrotherapy techniques from the Aromatherapy and Stimulating Solutions at least once a week.

6 Apply a weekly fake tan.

7 Have a weekly professional massage.

8 Try some of the professional anti-cellulite beauty treatments.

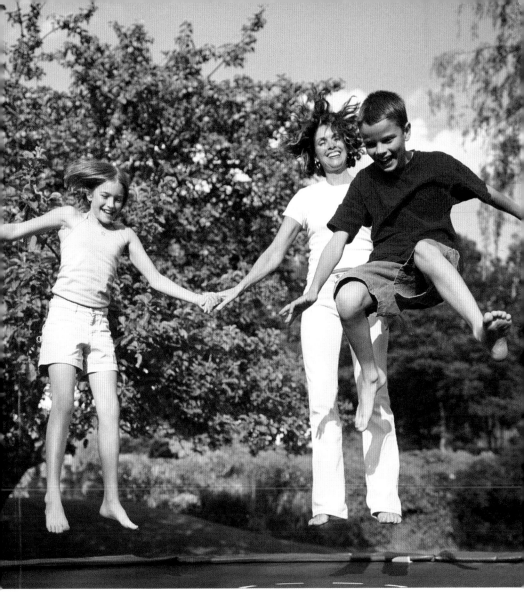

WHAT TO EXPECT

Like any change in health habits, following some of the cellulite Solutions may throw up some side effects, such as headaches as you cut down on caffeine. But don't panic – in each Solution where side effects or motivation may be an issue, there is plenty of advice on how to deal with any problems that may ensue.

One of the most important elements of this book is the section on Living the Anti-cellulite Life (see page 119). There is no point spending six weeks tackling your cellulite if you go back to all the habits that triggered it in the first place. The idea of this section is to discuss how to adapt your everyday life so that you are able to keep your cellulite under control.

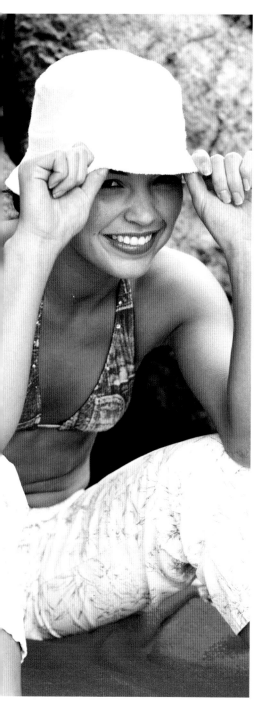

SIX WEEKS TO SUCCESS

I suggest the programme is used for six weeks. This is not a hard-and-fast rule, but it is the amount of time that will give results for the majority of people. It is also the minimum amount of time that people usually need to stop thinking of lifestyle changes as something new and strange, and make them a habit that becomes a natural part of their lives. But what can you realistically achieve in six weeks? If you follow the programme as directed, most people will:

- Lose at least 2.8 kg (6 lb) of excess weight (this will be less if you don't have excess weight to lose).
- Eliminate all excess fluid.
- Dramatically improve skin strength and condition.
- Boost muscle tone and lose inches from the hips and thighs.
- Boost circulation and lymph flow.
- Improve the detoxification capabilities of your body.
- Develop a healthier body image.

Exactly how much difference this will make to your cellulite depends on how your cellulite scores on the severity scale (see page 13). Obviously, someone suffering from severe cellulite is unlikely to have their cellulite disappear completely in six weeks, although you will notice a dramatic difference.

If at the end of six weeks you want to carry on with the Solutions, then do. If you have lost a lot of weight, however, check your BMI again (see page 15). If you are at a healthy weight, it is not advisable to follow the portion sizes suggested in the diet plan as these will lead to more weight loss. Read the advice on page 25, What if I don't need to lose weight?, to reveal how to adapt the diet. You will still be eating the same cellulite-busting foods, just more of them.

making time

It may seem daunting to actually find the time to put the plan into action. However, the difference between finding time and MAKING time is the key to getting results. Here are eight ideas that might work for you.

GET UP WHEN YOU WAKE UP
That extra 30 minutes you spend in bed doesn't really refresh you. By getting up when you wake up, you can reclaim 10–30 minutes a morning, enough to do your exercise programme or to give yourself an aromatherapy massage.

GO TO BED LATER
Not hours later, but spend 10 minutes before bed making your lunch for the next day and applying your anti-cellulite cream.

USE YOUR LUNCHBREAK
People who take a lunchbreak are more productive in the afternoon than those who work through. Use your lunchbreak for a short walk, a run or gym trip and you will feel even more energized.

TRAVEL TIME
If you are starting the plan as the days get lighter and warmer, is it possible for you to walk to or from work? If you live in a big city it may even be quicker for you to do so.

DEAD TIME
Make use of the time while the dinner's cooking, the kettle's coming up to the boil or the bath is running. There is nothing to say you can't spend this time skin brushing, applying fake tan or doing some exercise.

TELEVISION TIME
If kids or economy mean your evenings are normally spent in front of the TV, use this time instead for pamper nights using techniques from the beauty section. If you still want to watch the television, use advert breaks to rack up some exercise time, or even get an exercise bike in the sitting room.

KIDS' TIME
If you have children, finding time to go to the gym can be tricky, so involve the kids in your exercise plans. Older children can ride bikes while you jog, toddlers can enjoy the ride in a pushchair, or do activities you can all play – football in the park, rollerskating or frisbee in summer – you'll help their health too.

SOCIAL TIME
If evenings with friends always involve dinner and the pub, suggest something more active – bowling, salsa dancing classes, a nightclub, ice skating even – or go for pamper nights at the local salon. You'll see friends, but get your Solutions done too.

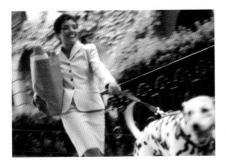

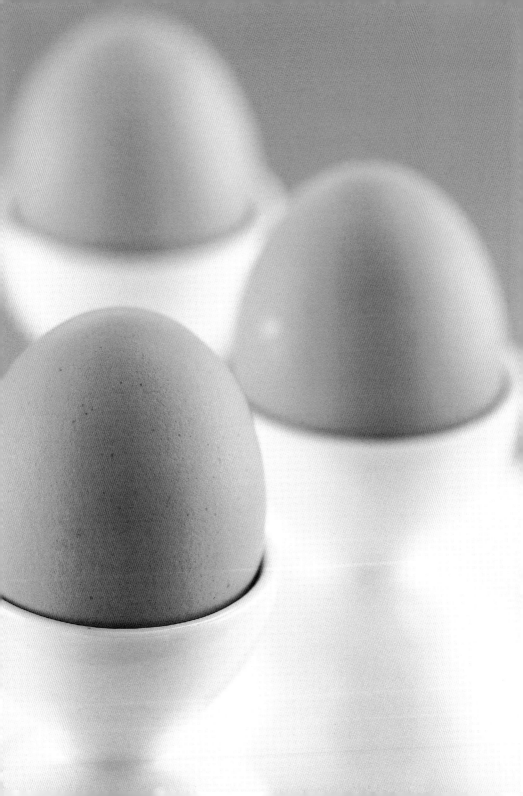

the
diet solution

The point of the Diet Solution is to harness the incredible powers of nutrients and use them to fight cellulite. Increasingly, dietary experts are discovering that what we eat greatly affects how healthy we are, and how healthy we look. It is estimated that roughly 40 per cent of cancers could be prevented if we just changed our diets, and that up to a million lives could be saved each year if we just took some dietary steps to protect our hearts. Even problems like failing eyesight, diabetes and strokes can be tackled through dietary measures. It is, therefore, no surprise that something as relatively simple and harmless as cellulite can be tackled through the foods we eat.

There is not one element of cellulite that cannot be positively influenced by diet – either through eliminating foods that contribute to its appearance, or by eating foods that help support the body in trying to get rid of it. On the Diet Solution, you will learn exactly what these foods are and how to eliminate those that need to go (without missing them). You will be shown how to increase the beneficial foods to flood your system with cellulite-fighting nutrients while still losing weight.

And the best thing about the Diet Solution is that even though you are on a diet, you won't be hungry, grumpy or bored of the foods you are eating. There are no starvation days, no just-juice days and no hunger headaches or grumbling stomachs. It isn't a matter of depriving your body, but fuelling it. There are some foods you need to cut out, but primarily you are aiming to feed your body to help you lose weight and fight fluid retention. You need to consume foods that supply the skin with antioxidant nutrients to fight free-radical damage, and foods that boost circulation or that stimulate the body's detoxification system and reduce pressure on the lymph. And finally, you want to add foods that provide high levels of nutrients to help fuel the process of skin regeneration. All this combines to fight cellulite at its source.

CONTENTS

losing weight

Combating cellulite through diet is a three-pronged approach that involves fighting fluid, fighting fat and fighting free radicals. While all of these are important, perhaps the most important for most of us is to lose weight to reduce those overfilled fat 'boxes'.

We gain fat when we eat more kilojoules/calories (collectively referred to as energy) than we use up in a day. For every 14,700 kJ or 3,500 kcal (calories) that we eat more than we burn, we put on about 0.5 kg (1 lb) in weight. We are genetically programmed to gain weight on our hips and thighs, which is why, when you go on a diet, it is always your breasts and stomach that lose the weight first and why it's harder to shift fat from your hips and thighs. But this doesn't mean you CAN'T lose weight from your bottom half. All it means is that you need to use more kilojoules/calories than you eat. Once your upper half has given up some fat, your bottom half will start responding.

HOW MUCH DO I NEED TO CUT OUT?

Just as 14,700 kJ (3,500 kcal) excess eaten means 0.5 kg (1 lb) added, if you reduce by 14,700 kJ (3,500 kcal) you will lose 0.5 kg (1 lb), but it is not a case of the more you cut out, the better. Our bodies are still living in Neanderthal times. They remember when food was hard to come by and if the supply dropped off, it could very well mean that famine was coming. So if you drastically cut your food intake, your body thinks you are going into starvation and slows down your metabolism, reducing the number of calories you burn.

Therefore, the rule for any diet is to cut only 2,100 kJ (500 kcal) from your recommended daily intake. If you do that every day you will lose 0.5 kg (1 lb) a week. This may sound slow, but it means you are more likely to be losing fat than muscle.

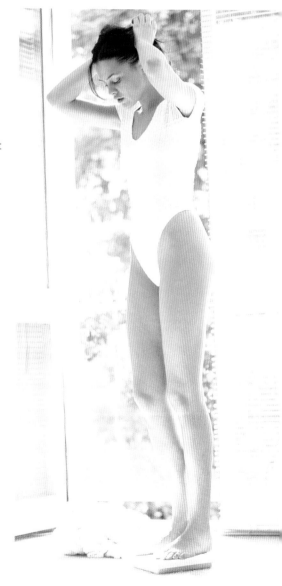

WHAT IS MY RECOMMENDED INTAKE?

To calculate how many kilojoules or calories you burn off in a day, and therefore how many you should be eating, you multiply your weight in pounds by 10 to get the number of calories you burn. If you are metrically minded, multiply your weight in kilograms by 92.4 to find your kilojoule expenditure. This is roughly how much energy you burn a day at rest, also known as your basal metabolic rate:

weight in pounds x 10 = calories burnt in a day
weight in kilos x 92.4 = kilojoules burnt in a day

Of course most of us don't spend all day lying on the sofa doing nothing – we move. Therefore, depending on how active you are, you need to multiply that figure further:

• If you have a sedentary job (office work) **multiply it by 1.3**
• If you have a moderately active job (shop worker, homemaker) **multiply it by 1.4**
• If you have a fairly active job (postperson, traffic warden) **multiply it by 1.5**
• If you have a very active job (builder, fitness trainer, courier) **multiply it by 1.7**

This gives the total amount of energy you burn on an average day. You should therefore be eating 2,100 kJ (500 kcal) less than this to lose 0.5 kg (1 lb) of weight a week. For example, if you weigh 70 kg (154 lb) and work in a shop, the calculation is as follows:

IN CALORIES
154 x 10 x 1.4 = 2,156 kcal per day burnt
2,156–500 = 1,656 kcal per day to eat on a diet

IN KILOJOULES
70 x 92.4 x 1.4 = 9,055 kJ per day burnt
9,055 2,100 − 6,955 kJ per day to eat on a diet

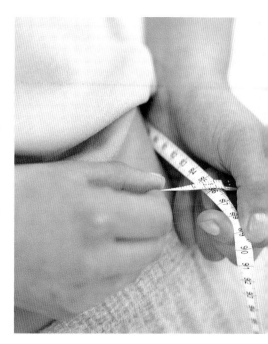

WHAT IF I DON'T NEED TO LOSE WEIGHT?

If you worked out your body mass index (BMI) on page 15 and found you were a healthy weight, losing fat won't help your cellulite – and in fact may cause you to lose lean muscle which could make the problem worse (muscle supports the fat layer, keeping it firmer and more stable). However, following the suggested foods and menu plans is still important as it will help you fight fluid and free-radical damage, but you need to increase the calories. The menu plans provide around 6,300 kJ (1,500 kcal) a day. If you don't need to lose weight, increase your portion sizes or add another snack so that your intake is equal to the amount you burn off each day.

SUCCESSFUL WEIGHT LOSS

Most of us dread diets and generally fail. Below are the reasons why we don't usually succeed, with an explanation of why this diet is different and why you will succeed this time.

you are hungry

This happens if you eat too little food or you don't eat foods that fill you up. This isn't the problem with this plan, as it is full of healthy, highly nutritious foods, which means you will be eating regularly and in large amounts. In fact, the plan is high in protein foods, which take the body a while to digest and fill you up for longer. If you do get hungry, however, try sniffing a little fennel oil (not if you are epileptic) to suppress your appetite.

you are fixated on food

The varied amounts of food and regular eating patterns on this diet should stop food fixation. But if you are really craving something, see the advice below.

you miss favourite foods

If at some point on the Diet Solution you're desperate for a favourite food (and it is the food you want, not a hug or a friend – see below), have a 420 kJ (100 kcal) portion of it. This would be a small packet of low-fat crisps, one chocolate biscuit, 25 g (1 oz) of boiled sweets or a 40 g (1½ oz) serving of low-fat ice cream. Knowing you can do this will often reduce cravings – and if it doesn't, could at least save you calories. Many of us try to fight cravings by snacking on huge quantities of a diet food, eating more calories than we would if we'd eaten a small portion of the thing we really want.

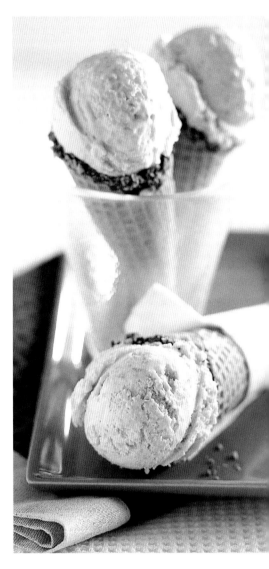

you think you're going to fail

As soon as you eat something that's not on the plan, you immediately think you have failed. That's not true – one high-fat meal does not make you fat, nor does it stop you losing weight. It is only the second, third or fourth that do that. If you slip off the programme, don't panic and give up, just go back to it.

you eat when you are stressed, tired or bored

Many of us eat to tackle negative emotions. If you find yourself craving sugar or starchy foods, ask yourself if you really want those – or if you need a hug, some company or a day off. Then set about getting what you really want rather than suppressing the emotion with food.

THE ENERGY IN SOME COMMON FOODS

	kJ	kcal
Milk (semi-skimmed, per 600 ml (1 pint)	820	195
Nuts (per 25 g/1 oz)	760–800	180–190
Potato (per 175 g/6 oz)	630	150
Can of soft drink (non-diet)	550	130
Olive oil (per tablespoon)	525	125
Cheese (hard – per 25 g/1 oz)	460	110
Muesli (no added sugar, per 25 g/1 oz)	460	110
Cornflakes (per 25 g/1 oz)	440	105
Avocado (per half)	420	100
Fruit juice (per 250 ml/8 fl oz)	420	100
Rice (per 25 g/1 oz dry weight)	420	100
Pasta (per 25 g/1 oz dry weight)	420	100
Bran flakes (per 25 g/1 oz)	380	90
Banana	380	90
Bacon (per grilled back rasher)	360	85
Wine (per 125 ml/4 fl oz glass)	354	85
Eggs (each)	340	80
Bread (per slice)	340	80
Lamb chop (per 25 g/1 oz, fat removed)	260	62
Apple	250	60
Beef (per 25 g/1 oz steak or roast)	210	50
Orange	210	50
Chicken (per 25 g/1 oz, skin removed)	135	32
Rice cakes (each)	125	30
Shellfish (per 25 g/1 oz without shells)	105–125	25–30
Fish (fresh, per 25 g/1 oz)	85–125	20–30
Tofu (per 25 g/1 oz)	105	25
Cottage cheese (low-fat – per 25 g/1 oz)	90	22
Beans (per 25 g/1 oz raw)	85	20
Sugar (per teaspoon)	70	17
Yogurt (low-fat, per tablespoon)	42	10
Watermelon (per 25 g/1 oz)	38	9
Vegetables (green, per 25 g/1 oz)	17–34	4–8
Berries (per 25 g/1 oz)	30	7
Coffee (no milk)	0	0
Tea (no milk)	0	0

cellulite sin foods

Diet is a great remedy for cellulite – but what we eat can also be a major cause of the problem. While many foods have the ability to do us good, others can cause fluid retention, skin damage, poor circulation and even slow, sluggish lymph flow. These are obviously foods that you should cut out completely or at least significantly reduce during the Diet Solution. Here are the top seven.

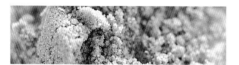

SUGAR As well as the fact that sugar usually comes packed inside high-fat, high-calorie foods, scientists at State University in Buffalo have discovered that the amount of free radicals in your system increases by 140 per cent after eating 1,260 kJ (300 kcal) of sugar. This alone is bad news for your collagen, but sugar also causes collagen to harden, making the septa pull down on the skin and the fat more visible. This hardening can also occur in the arteries and blood vessels, and slow circulation. Try to cut sugary foods from your diet completely.

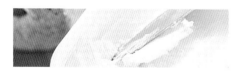

SATURATED FATS AND TRANSFATS
If you want to gain fat, eat fat. At 38 kJ (9 kcal) per 25 g (1 oz) (compared to less than half that for carbohydrates or protein), it's the easiest way to consume more than you need. Also, saturated fats (found in animal products like meat, butter and full-fat dairy) and altered vegetable fats called transfats or hydrogenated fats (found in margarines and spreads) double free-radical levels almost straight away. Aim to keep the fat content of your diet under 30 per cent of your daily energy intake, with no more than 10 per cent from saturated fats.

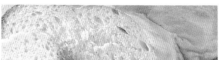

REFINED CARBOHYDRATES These are white sugars, flours, rice, pasta and bread. They are the staple part of our diet for most of us, but they could also trigger weight gain. Refined carbohydrates cause a sudden flood of glucose, the sugar we need for fuel, to enter our systems. The body tries to balance things by releasing insulin, which pushes the glucose into the body's fat stores. This constant see-sawing causes some people (possibly up to 25 per cent of us) to become less sensitive to insulin, which means the body needs to produce more to get results – increasing the amount of fat we store. To avoid its effects, switch the majority of refined foods to their wholefood versions – this means brown rice, wholemeal wheat-free pasta, rye and pumpernickel breads or oatcakes, and bran-based cereals.

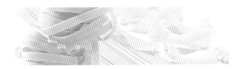

WHEAT As discussed on page 16, food intolerances can cause cellulite, and wheat is one of the worst culprits. The main reason is that food intolerances occur when you are overexposed to a food, and wheat is found in bread, pasta, pizza, pastries, biscuits and cakes and is also a common food additive (it is often found in stock cubes, ready-made sauces and sausages, to name but a few). To add to this problem, today's wheat contains high levels of natural chemicals called lectins, and many types of lectin are actually toxic to our bodies. On the Diet Solution, you are going to skip all wheat-heavy foods.

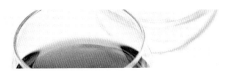

ALCOHOL Like coffee, alcohol is not banned on the Diet Solution, but it needs to be handled with care. In small doses alcohol dilates blood vessels and thins the blood. However, after one drink this changes and fat levels in the blood start to increase, slowing circulation. Alcohol also creates high numbers of free radicals in the system and boosts oestrogen levels (which may encourage fluid retention). Finally, alcohol switches off the system in the stomach that allows you to absorb vitamins, including fat burners like vitamin C, zinc and calcium. On the Diet Solution try not to drink more than one alcoholic drink a day.

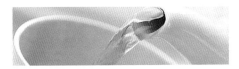

CAFFEINE In most anti-cellulite plans, caffeine is totally banned – that's not the case in this one, as small doses can boost circulation and speed up the metabolism. If you consume more than one cup, however, this balance changes and the arteries start to stiffen, slowing circulation. On top of this, the increase in your metabolism could be cancelled out by your growing need for sugary treats, as high doses of caffeine cause sudden rises and falls in blood-sugar levels. Aim to limit caffeine intake to one cup of tea, coffee or cola every three hours, and no more than two or three a day.

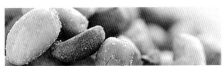

SALTY FOODS Fluid levels in our bodies are governed by two minerals: sodium and potassium. When the two of these are in balance, so is the level of fluid in our bodies – but often they are out of balance. Most of us eat too much salt in crisps, peanuts, bacon and ready meals, and when this happens the body tries to dilute it by retaining fluid in the tissues, compounding the cellulite problem. The World Health Organization recommends we eat no more than 5 g (1/4 oz) of salt (sodium) per day. Aim for this amount while you are on the Diet Solution – read labels carefully and don't add salt at the table or while cooking.

top 20 anti-cellulite foods

If you have looked at the cellulite sin foods on the previous pages, you may be wondering what you can eat on the Diet Solution. The answer is anything that isn't one of the seven cellulite sins. If you want to maximize effects, however, try to focus on the following foods, which actually have cellulite-fighting properties.

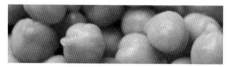

BEANS AND PULSES Full of fibre, but also providing protein, beans are a great vegetarian choice on the anti-cellulite plan. Also include:
Calcium Important for fighting body fat
Potassium Helps to fight fluid retention

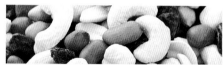

NUTS Another high-protein choice, nuts are also full of nutrients. Just two Brazil nuts provide your recommended daily intake of the vital antioxidant selenium. Also include:
Vitamin E Improves circulation as well as skin
Monounsaturated fat This helps the body burn fat

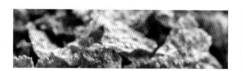

BRAN AND OAT CEREALS Breakfast is the most important meal of the day for cellulite sufferers. Those who eat cereal regularly weigh an average of 4 kg (8 lb) less than those who don't. Also include:
Fibre An excellent fat-buster and keeps energy levels up all day
Antioxidants A bowl of bran or oat cereal contains as many as a bowl of plums

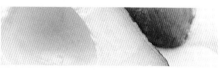

AVOCADOS They may be high in calories, but they are packed with essential fatty acids, which improve the health of the skin and circulation and may also help your body burn fat.
Also include:
Vitamin E Vital for healthy skin
Beta sitosterol This fibre helps fight cholesterol and may improve circulation

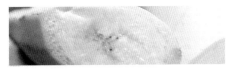

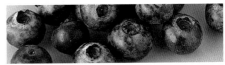

BANANAS An excellent booster for blood vessels, bananas can't be beaten for healthy circulation and are a great snack at any time of day. Also include:
Potassium Fights fluid retention
Vitamin B6 Another fluid fighter
Magnesium Helps fight stress and its associated weight gain

BERRIES Berries are among the top antioxidant foods, counteracting the sugar, fats and other pollutants that damage skin and create the orange-peel effect. Also include:
Vitamin C A powerful detoxifier and helps strengthen the skin
Gamma linoleic acid Found in blackberries, this helps certain types of body fat burn more calories

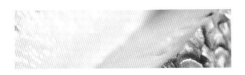

PINEAPPLE Pineapple has an anti-inflammatory action in the body, which may help fight fluid retention and aid in the healing of damaged collagen fibres. Also includes:
Vitamin C Potentially the most important cellulite-fighting vitamin
Protein digestors Help the body use this vital food group

SHOULD I GO ORGANIC?
Non-organic foods can contain traces of pesticides and fertilizers that are toxic. The body pushes these into the fat stores where they do less damage, then floods the stores with water to dilute these toxins, exacerbating the cellulite problem. If you don't go organic, at least peel or scrub all fruit and vegetables before eating them.

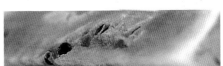

PEARS Extremely detoxifying, pears can help reduce the effects of pollutants in the system, aiding the lymph.
Also include:
Iodine This mineral helps stimulate a sluggish metabolism
Fibre Also a weight-loss aid and vital for healthy digestion
Potassium To help fight fluid

WATERMELON Fluid-filled foods fight fluid retention – and watermelon contains a glass of · water per slice. Also includes:
Lycopene A vital antioxidant
Potassium Fights fluid retention by keeping fluid levels in the body balanced
Fibre good for circulation

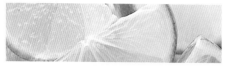

CITRUS FRUITS One medium orange provides 80mg of vitamin C, twice the recommended daily intake for adults, vital for the building of collagen. Also include:
Methoxylated bioflavonoids Improve circulation and strengthen capillaries
B vitamins Good for energy and circulation

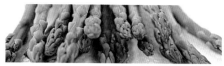

ASPARAGUS Asparagus is a top cellulite-buster because it strengthens veins and capillaries and controls blood pressure. Also includes:
Glutathione A detoxifying enzyme and free-radical fighter
Vitamin A, vitamin C Help to strengthen the skin
B vitamins Create healthy circulation and lymph

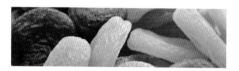

DRIED FRUITS Fruits high in potassium, such as prunes, figs and apricots, help regulate fluid. Also include:
Fibre Good for regulating bowel movements, reducing risk of food intolerances and toxic overload
Zinc Vital for fat burning

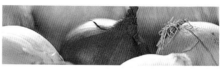

ONIONS An important ingredient for many meals, onions are easy to incorporate into your everyday diet and excellent for busting cellulite. Also include:
Sulphur Reduces free-radical damage
Vitamin C Antioxidant that helps build collagen
Vitamin E Protects cell membranes and prevents fats being oxidized

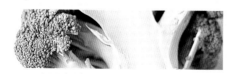

BROCCOLI Contains an ingredient called alpha lipoic acid that prevents the hardening of collagen caused by sugar. Also includes:
Selenium Improves the action of vitamins C, E and beta carotene
Calcium One broccoli portion gives 10 per cent of your recommended daily calcium intake

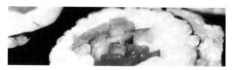

SEA VEGETABLES High in minerals, sea vegetables like nori and kelp are also full of antioxidants that detoxify and refresh tired skin. Also include:
Iodine Maximizes calorie burning by helping to speed metabolism
Ligans Powerful detoxifiers that combat the effects of toxins, such as pollution, radiation and free-radical damage
Potassium Prevents fluid retention

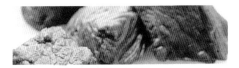

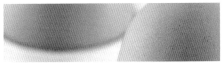

BEEF (LEAN) One of the highest dietary sources of a fat-burning nutrient called conjugated linoleic acid. Also includes:
Iron Vital for boosting energy, particularly during exercise
Protein To help fight fluid retention

EGGS In the body, eggs create a sulphur-based compound, which helps detoxify alcohol and other toxins, reducing the amount of free radicals they can cause. Also include:
Protein A good fill-up food for vegetarians
Vitamin A Egg yolks are a great source of this antioxidant

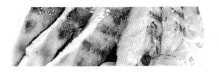

POULTRY A good low-fat source of protein, just remember to remove the skin and stick to white, not dark meat.
Also includes:
Zinc The body needs this to burn fat
B vitamins Help boost energy

A WORD ABOUT EGGS
Although eggs contain essential nutrients and help to detoxify the body, they also contain cholesterol, so be careful not to eat them too often.

Pregnant women, young children and the elderly should avoid eating raw or undercooked eggs.

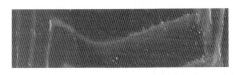

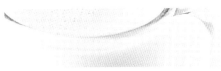

OILY FISH Salmon, tuna, mackerel, trout, herrings, sardines and bass are quick and easy to prepare as well as being low in fat and high in anti-cellulite proteins and minerals. Also includes:
Essential fatty acids These help build healthy, firm skin
Prostaglandins Help regulate fluid, support blood vessels and promote circulation

SEMI-SKIMMED MILK AND LOW-FAT CHEESES Dairy products are the richest source of fat-burning calcium available and are therefore vital in combating cellulite. They can cause food intolerances, however (see page 16). Also include:
Conjugated linoleic acid Increases fat loss and muscle gain and is believed to have antioxidant properties

getting maximum benefit

We have already discussed the three main premises of the Diet Solution: eating 2,100 kJ (500 kcal) per day less than your basal metabolic rate (see page 24); avoiding the seven cellulite sin foods (see page 28); and focusing on beneficial anti-cellulite foods (see page 30). However, there are four further rules that will maximize the effects of the Diet Solution and get the best results.

1 EAT FIVE PORTIONS OF FRUIT AND VEGETABLES A DAY

Fruit and vegetables are packed with a multitude of antioxidant nutrients, but in particular supply the vital nutrients beta carotene (which the body converts to vitamin A) and vitamin C (which our skin needs to help trigger the process of regeneration), plus essential minerals that we need to trigger fat burning. Five portions is the minimum amount that is likely to supply optimum levels of these nutrients – with a portion being a 250 g (8 oz) slice of large fruits like watermelon, 2 tablespoons of small fruits like berries or any vegetables, or one medium fruit such as an apple or orange. Many people think that eating five portions a day is tricky, but it doesn't have to be. Just remember these four points:

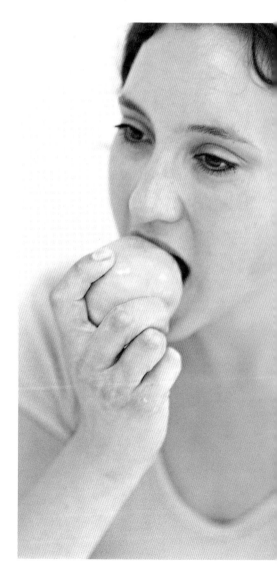

- Fresh, frozen or tinned fruit or vegetables all count.
- Focus on the 'one meal, one portion' rule. If five a day sounds like too much, instead focus on achieving one portion with every meal or snack you eat.
- If you don't think you like fruit and vegetables, experiment with new varieties to find ones you do like. While the foods mentioned in the Top 20 will have the best effects against cellulite, any fruit or vegetable will supply some levels of vital antioxidants. Try sweet potatoes, papaya, mangetouts, lychees, rocket or red leaf lettuce, red cabbage (not white), or baby carrots instead of normal ones.

- Experiment with new ways of serving them. Instead of boiling vegetables, try roasting, stir-frying or steaming them – you can even grill or purée fruit to change its taste or texture. And there's no logical reason why you can't eat fruit with meals instead of vegetables: many great salads add servings of citrus fruit or apples alongside white cabbage or celery, for example. Or just serve a huge fruit salad instead of a savoury version.

2 EAT SOME LEAN PROTEIN AT LEAST THREE TIMES A DAY

Protein contains a substance called albumin that helps absorb excess fluid in the tissues of the body – if fluid retention is part of your problem, this will help. Protein also keeps your blood sugar steady longer than eating a meal of carbohydrates alone. This prevents blood-sugar swings that can trigger sugar cravings and hunger pangs – both of which make some diet plans too hard to follow. Lean proteins include fish, poultry, shellfish, low-fat dairy, beans, pulses, lean cuts of red meat with all fat removed, plus vegetarian proteins like tofu, Quorn or TVP.

3 EAT SOMETHING FIVE OR SIX TIMES A DAY

Eating more often can actually boost your weight-loss potential, as every time you eat your body has to burn energy to digest the food. In fact, 10 per cent of the energy you burn each day occurs during digestion and this boost to your metabolism lasts a few hours. Keep nibbling on fruit, vegetables or other low-fat snacks and your metabolism will be fired up round the clock.

However, one of the biggest mistakes people make when eating five or six times a day is to eat too much. We are used to eating three big meals a day, and shrinking portions can create 'psychological hunger' where you start to crave food even though your body doesn't need it. Stick to small meals, however, and pile on fresh fruit and vegetables to fool your brain into

SIX-WEEK EATING PLAN

So what do all these rules and pointers mean you are going to be eating in practice? Over the next few pages you will find a three-week eating plan, which you will complete twice throughout the six weeks of the overall plan – or just use as a guide to help you plan your own meals following the energy count chart on page 27. It supplies all the anti-cellulite foods you need, while eliminating the seven cellulite sin foods almost completely. It supplies roughly 6,300 kj (1,500 kcal) a day, which is the amount required by an average 70 kg (11 stone) woman in a sedentary job if she wants to lose 0.5 kg (1 lb) a week. If you weigh less than this, but still need to lose weight, decrease portion sizes slightly to drop calories (but don't skip any meals as this will reduce your calorie-burning potential). If you are heavier than this, likewise adapt your portion sizes accordingly. If you don't need to lose weight, see the box on page 25.

thinking there's more food (without adding extra calories). If your brain is telling you it is too small an amount of food, just remind yourself that there's another snack along in two hours.

4 DRINK LOTS OF CAFFEINE-FREE FLUIDS

Every day on the diet, aim to drink at least 1 litre (1¾ pints) of water. You can also drink unlimited herbal teas – see the Supplement Solution for suggestions of those that could actually increase the diet's effects.

six-week eating plan: weeks 1&4

The following pages give you a six-week eating plan that includes the top anti-cellulite foods, and omits the seven sin foods as far as possible. Remember that if you do not need to lose weight, you must increase the quantities to give you more calories per day (see page 25).

	cellulite fighters	breakfast	snack
DAY 1	*banana, berries, bran, broccoli, citrus, dairy, eggs, nuts, onions, pears, poultry*	25 g (1 oz) bran cereal with 250 ml (8 fl oz) of semi-skimmed milk. Add 1 chopped banana and a handful of blackcurrants	3 satsumas 40 g (1½ oz) Brazil nuts
DAY 2	*asparagus, avocado, banana, berries, dairy, dried fruit, eggs, oily fish, sea vegetables, watermelon*	2 slices of rye toast topped with 1 mashed banana Fruit Smoothie (see page 42)	1 small pot of low-fat yogurt mixed with 3 chopped dried apricots
DAY 3	*avocado, broccoli, citrus, dairy, eggs, oats, onions, pears, pineapple, pulses*	1 boiled egg 2 slices of rye toast with a little low-fat spread 1 glass of orange juice (preferably calcium-enriched)	50 g (2 oz) low-fat edam cheese on 2 oatcakes topped with a sliced tomato
DAY 4	*asparagus, banana, beans, beef, berries, citrus, dairy, eggs, nuts, onions, pears, pineapple, pulses*	Fruit Plate (see page 43)	1 slice of rye toast topped with 1 teaspoon peanut butter 1 pear
DAY 5	*asparagus, berries, citrus, dairy, dried fruit, nuts, oats, onions, pineapple, pulses*	Pumpkin Seed and Apricot Muesli (see page 42) Half a grapefruit	2 slices of pineapple
DAY 6	*banana, broccoli, citrus, dairy, eggs, nuts, oily fish, onions, pears*	1 mango, halved and grilled for 2 minutes 75 g (3 oz) low-fat cottage cheese 1 slice of rye toast	1 banana 4 Brazil nuts
DAY 7	*asparagus, avocado, banana, beans, berries, citrus, dairy, eggs, nuts, oats, onions, pears*	2 oatcakes topped with 1 mashed banana Handful of blueberries	2 celery sticks dipped in 1 teaspoon of peanut butter

lunch	snack	dinner
250 g (8 oz) jacket potato topped with either 100 g (3½ oz) drained tuna in brine, 1 tablespoon of lemon juice and a little chopped onion; or 100 g (3½ oz) low-fat cottage cheese with chives Serve with salad of rocket, red pepper, celery and alfalfa sprouts	2 crispbreads topped with 2 handfuls of sliced strawberries 1 pear	125 g (4 oz) grilled chicken breast; or Lemon Grass and Tofu Nuggets (see page 48) Tomato Salsa (see page 42) 100 g (3½ oz) sweet potato, baked in its skin Unlimited boiled or steamed green beans, broccoli and carrots 1 small pot of low-fat yogurt
6 pieces of Rice Ball Sushi (see page 45) 1 bowl of Miso Soup, instant or home-made (see page 44)	Large slice of watermelon	100 g (3½ oz) grilled trout fillet; or a two-egg omelette with sliced mushrooms 100 g (3½ oz) new potatoes 5 asparagus spears and 1 sliced tomato 1 small pot of low-fat yogurt
Chicken, Avocado and Mango Salad (see page 45); vegetarians can omit the chicken and use a whole avocado	1 pear 1 slice of pineapple 1 small pot of low-fat yogurt	Braised Lentils with Mushrooms and Gremolata (see page 47) Steamed green beans, broccoli and spinach
1 small can of tomato soup 50 g (2 oz) shop-bought hummus; or Fava (see page 43) Carrot, celery, spring onion, cucumber and red pepper sticks for dipping	1 orange 1 apple	Hot Thai Beef Salad (see page 55); or Watercress, Mushroom and Asparagus Frittata (see page 46) 1 banana, baked in its skin until soft, served with 1 tablespoon of low-fat yogurt
150 g (5 oz) jacket potato topped with 125 g (4 oz) low-fat coleslaw Unlimited salad of alfalfa sprouts, red peppers and beetroot	1 small pot of low-fat yogurt Handful of raspberries	Colourful Kebabs (see page 50) 75 g (3 oz) brown rice, boiled Steamed asparagus Tomato Salsa (see page 42)
Potato, Celery and Apple Salad (see page 46) 1 pear	1 small pot of low-fat yogurt 1 orange	Poached Salmon with Hot Basil Sauce (see page 51); or Eggs Benedict (see page 48) Unlimited boiled or steamed carrots, broccoli and dark green cabbage
Salad Niçoise (see page 45)	Fruit Smoothie (see page 42)	Aubergine Towers (see page 47) 1 small can of baked beans 2 pears, chopped and topped with 2 tablespoons of low-fat yogurt and 1 teaspoon of honey

DAY 1

DAY 2

DAY 3

DAY 4

DAY 5

DAY 6

DAY 7

six-week eating plan: weeks 2&5

	cellulite fighters	breakfast	snack
DAY 1	asparagus, berries, citrus, dairy, dried fruit, eggs, oily fish, onions, pears, poultry	1 poached egg 1 slice of rye toast 1 glass of orange juice (preferably calcium-enriched)	25 g (1 oz) dried cranberries 1 pear
DAY 2	avocado, banana, beans, beef, broccoli, citrus, oats, oily fish, onions, pears, sea vegetables	2 slices of rye toast 1 small can of baked beans (no added salt) 1 glass of orange juice (preferably calcium-enriched) 1 satsuma	1 pear 1 banana
DAY 3	asparagus, banana, bran, broccoli, citrus, dairy, dried fruit, eggs, oily fish, onions, pears	25 g (1 oz) bran flakes with 250 ml (8 fl oz) semi-skimmed milk, topped with 1 pear, sliced, and 25 g (1 oz) raisins	50 g (2 oz) low-fat cottage cheese 3 celery sticks for dipping
DAY 4	avocado, banana, beans, citrus, eggs, oily fish, onions, poultry, watermelon	2 slices of rye toast topped with 1 mashed banana	Fruit Smoothie (see page 42)
DAY 5	beans, beef, berries, broccoli, citrus, dairy, dried fruit, nuts, oats, onions, pulses	Pumpkin Seed and Apricot Muesli (see page 42) 1 handful of strawberries	50 g (2 oz) low-fat cottage cheese 2 satsumas
DAY 6	asparagus, avocado, banana, berries, broccoli, citrus, dairy, dried fruit, oats, oily fish, onions	Fruit Smoothie (see page 42) 2 crispbreads topped with 1 teaspoon of honey	3 celery sticks 75 g (3 oz) tuna mixed with lemon juice
DAY 7	asparagus, banana, berries, broccoli, citrus, dairy, dried fruit, nuts, onions, pineapple, poultry, watermelon	Fruit Plate (see page 43)	1 slice of rye toast topped with one teaspoonful of peanut butter

lunch	snack	dinner	
Asparagus Guacamole (see page 43) Carrot, cucumber and celery sticks for dipping A few cherry tomatoes Carrot and Sage Soup (see page 44)	2 crispbreads topped with 50 g (2 oz) tuna, or 25 g (1 oz) low-fat edam cheese 2 tablespoons of Tomato Salsa (see page 42)	Cranberry Chicken Stir-fry with Ginger (see page 53); replace chicken with tofu for a vegetarian alternative 75 g (3 oz) brown rice, boiled	DAY 1
5 pieces of Rice Ball Sushi (see page 45) 1 bowl of Miso Soup, instant or home-made (see page 44)	2 oatcakes topped with half an avocado and some slices of red pepper	125 g (4 oz) lean roast beef; or 1 large grilled mushroom topped with Ratatouille (see page 43) 150 g (5 oz) jacket potato Unlimited green beans, dark green cabbage and broccoli	DAY 2
150 g (5 oz) jacket potato topped with Tomato Salsa (see page 42) and 75 g (3 oz) tuna in brine, drained, or 50 g (2 oz) grated low-fat cheese 1 glass of orange juice (preferably calcium-enriched)	2 handfuls of strawberries 1 banana	Eggs Benedict (see page 48) 150 g (5 oz) potato, boiled and mashed with a little semi-skimmed milk Unlimited steamed asparagus and broccoli 1 small pot of low-fat yogurt	DAY 3
Bean Salad (see page 46) 125 g (4 oz) shredded roast chicken breast; or 1 boiled egg Large green salad	Large slice of watermelon	125 g (4 oz) grilled tuna steak; or Lemon Grass and Tofu Nuggets (see page 48) 75 g (3 oz) boiled new potatoes with fresh mint Half an avocado Tomato Salsa (see page 42)	DAY 4
Open sandwich made from 1 slice of rye bread spread with Asparagus Guacamole (see page 43), alfalfa sprouts, sliced tomato and yellow peppers	1 small can of tomato soup 2 handfuls of blueberries 6 almonds	Beef and Broccoli with Oyster Sauce (see page 55); or Cabbage, Beetroot and Apple Sauté (see page 50) 75 g (3 oz) brown rice, boiled	DAY 5
Half an avocado filled with 50 g (2 oz) cooked peeled prawns or 4 tablespoons of Tomato Salsa (see page 42)	Salad of rocket, red pepper and artichoke hearts 2 oatcakes topped with 1 mashed banana	Anglo-Indian Curry (see page 51) 50 g (2 oz) brown rice, boiled Unlimited steamed asparagus	DAY 6
Watercress, Mushroom and Asparagus Frittata (see page 46) 1 glass of orange juice (preferably calcium-enriched)	Large slice of watermelon	Chicken, Squash and Sweet Potato Tagine (see page 52); or Aubergine Towers (see page 47) Unlimited steamed broccoli and green beans	DAY 7

six-week eating plan: weeks 3&6

	cellulite fighters	breakfast	snack
DAY 1	asparagus, avocado, banana, beef, broccoli, citrus, dairy, onions, pears, poultry, watermelon	1 slice of rye toast topped with 50 g (2 oz) grated low-fat edam cheese and 2 sliced tomatoes, grilled 1 pear	Large slice of watermelon
DAY 2	avocado, beans, berries, citrus, dairy, dried fruit, oats, oily fish, onions, pears, pineapple	Oat-based porridge, made with water topped with 1 chopped pear and 25 g (1 oz) sultanas Fava (see page 43)	Cucumber and carrot sticks for dipping
DAY 3	avocado, banana, beans, citrus, dairy, dried fruit, eggs, nuts, oats, oily fish, onions	Pumpkin Seed and Apricot Muesli (see page 42)	1 small pot of low-fat yogurt 1 banana
DAY 4	banana, citrus, dairy, dried fruit, eggs, oily fish, onions, poultry, watermelon	1 egg, scrambled with a little semi-skimmed milk 50 g (2 oz) smoked salmon; or 1 slice of rye toast Half a grapefruit	Large slice of watermelon 1 small pot of low-fat yogurt
DAY 5	asparagus, banana, beef, bran, citrus, dairy, eggs, oily fish, onions, pears, pulses	25 g (1 oz) bran cereal topped with 250 ml (8 fl oz) semi-skimmed milk and 1 chopped banana	50 g (2 oz) shop-bought tzatziki Carrot, celery and cucumber sticks for dipping
DAY 6	berries, broccoli, citrus, dairy, eggs, nuts, onions, pears, watermelon	1 boiled egg 2 slices of rye toast topped with a little low-fat spread 2 handfuls of strawberries or raspberries	25 g (1 oz) almonds 1 pear
DAY 7	berries, broccoli, citrus, dairy, dried fruit, eggs, nuts, onions, pineapple, poultry	Omelette made with the whites of 2 eggs plus 1 whole egg and filled with mixed berries 1 glass of orange juice (preferably calcium-enriched)	Half an apple topped with 1 teaspoon of peanut butter

lunch	snack	dinner	
Chicken, Avocado and Mango Salad (see page 45); vegetarians can omit the chicken and use a whole avocado	1 banana 1 small pot of low-fat yogurt	125 g (4 oz) lean steak or Quorn steak, grilled 125 g (4 oz) new potatoes Tomato Salsa (see page 42) Unlimited steamed asparagus and broccoli	DAY 1
150 g (5 oz) jacket potato topped with either 100 g (3½ oz) drained tuna in brine mixed with 1 tablespoon of lemon juice and a little chopped onion; or 100 g (3½ oz) low-fat cottage cheese with chives Unlimited salad of rocket, red pepper, celery and alfalfa sprouts	1 slice of pineapple 2 handfuls of strawberries	Mexican Soup with Avocado Salsa (see page 50) 2 slices of rye bread	DAY 2
125 g (4 oz) cooked peeled prawns; or 1 boiled egg Half an avocado Large salad of lettuce, radish, tomato and yellow pepper	2 crispbreads topped with Fava (see page 43)	125 g (4 oz) grilled sardines; or 2 courgettes, halved and grilled until soft, then topped with 25 g (1 oz) low-fat feta cheese Bean Salad (see page 46) 1 glass of orange juice (preferably calcium-enriched)	DAY 3
Potato, Celery and Apple Salad (see page 46)	1 slice of rye toast topped with 1 mashed banana	Cranberry Chicken Stir-fry with Ginger (see page 53); replace chicken with tofu for a vegetarian alternative 50 g (2 oz) brown rice, boiled	DAY 4
Salad Niçoise (see page 45)	1 orange 1 pear	Beef Tacos (see page 53); or Braised Lentils with Mushrooms and Gremolata (see page 47) Bowl of strawberries and raspberries drizzled with 1 teaspoon of honey	DAY 5
150 g (5 oz) jacket potato topped with 125 g (4 oz) Ratatouille (see page 43) Large salad of shredded white cabbage, grated carrot and red onions	1 glass of orange juice 1 large slice of watermelon 25 g (1 oz) low-fat cheese	Colourful Kebabs (see page 50) Tomato Salsa (see page 42) 50 g (2 oz) brown rice, boiled Unlimited steamed broccoli	DAY 6
Open sandwich made with 1 slice of rye bread spread with a little mustard, 125 g (4 oz) of lean roast turkey or 2 slices of low-fat cheese, and slices of tomato, alfalfa sprouts and red pepper	2 slices of pineapple 1 small pot of low-fat yogurt	Anglo-Indian Curry (see page 51)	DAY 7

recipes

The following recipes feature in the six-week diet plan and are packed with cellulite-busting ingredients. Delicious and nutritious, they will be enjoyed by the whole family, whether fighting cellulite or not.

pumpkin seed and apricot muesli
MAKES **2 SERVINGS**

50 g (2 oz) rolled jumbo oats
1 tablespoon sultanas
1 tablespoon pumpkin seeds
1 tablespoon chopped almonds
25 g (1 oz) dried apricots, chopped
2 tablespoons orange juice
2 small eating apples, peeled and grated
3 tablespoons semi-skimmed milk

1 Place the oats, sultanas, pumpkin seeds, almonds and apricots in a bowl with the orange juice.

2 Add the grated apple and stir. Top with the milk and serve immediately.

fruit smoothie
MAKES **1 SERVING**

2 tablespoons blueberries or blackcurrants
2 tablespoons strawberries
250 ml (8 fl oz) orange juice
1 banana

Place all the ingredients in a blender or food processor and blend until smooth.

tomato salsa
MAKES **3–4 SERVINGS**

A healthy, vibrant salsa that will brighten up many different dishes. Serve with jacket potatoes, plain grilled meat, fish or vegetables for a fat-free burst of flavour.

1 red onion, finely chopped
425 g (14 oz) vine-ripened tomatoes, deseeded and chopped
2 garlic cloves, crushed
15 g (1/2 oz) fresh coriander, mint or parsley, chopped
pepper

Mix together all the ingredients in a bowl and season with pepper.

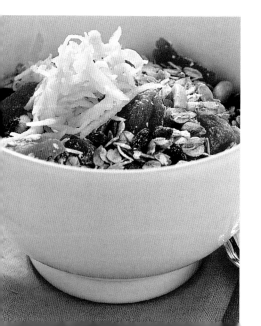

fruit plate
MAKES **1 SERVING**

2 slices of pineapple
1/2 mango
1 banana, chopped
2 kiwi fruits
2 tablespoons strawberries
1 small pot of low-fat natural yogurt

Arrange all the fruits on a plate and spoon the yogurt on top.

fava
MAKES **4 SERVINGS**

This puréed bean paste is similar to hummus, but is made with yellow split peas.

50 g (2 oz) yellow split peas, rinsed
2 tablespoons extra-virgin olive oil
1 small garlic clove, crushed
1 tablespoon lemon juice
1/2 teaspoon ground cumin
1/2 teaspoon mustard powder
pinch of cayenne pepper
pepper

to garnish:
1 tablespoon chopped parsley
1 tablespoon chopped red pepper

1 Put the split peas in a saucepan and add enough cold water to cover the peas by about 2.5 cm (1 inch). Bring to the boil and simmer over a low heat, stirring frequently, for 30–35 minutes until all the water is absorbed and the peas are cooked. Leave to cool slightly.

2 Place the peas in a liquidizer with all the remaining ingredients, season to taste, and process until smooth.

3 Transfer to a serving dish and sprinkle with the parsley and red pepper.

ratatouille
MAKES **4 SERVINGS**

1 tablespoon olive oil
2 onions, chopped
2 red peppers, chopped
1 green pepper, chopped
2 garlic cloves, chopped
3 courgettes, chopped
400 g (13 oz) can of chopped tomatoes
handful of basil leaves, chopped
salt and pepper

1 Heat the oil in a large saucepan. Add the onions and cook over a low heat for 10 minutes without browning.

2 Add the peppers and continue to cook for a further 20 minutes without browning. Stir in the garlic and courgettes, fry for a few minutes, then add the tomatoes.

3 Turn up the heat and cook until the liquid has reduced and the vegetables are tender. Season with pepper and just a little salt, then stir in the basil. Serve hot or cold. Any leftovers can be frozen successfully.

asparagus guacamole
MAKES **1 SERVING**

75 g (3 oz) asparagus
1 tablespoon low-fat crème fraîche
small piece of onion, finely chopped
1 tomato, chopped
splash of lemon juice

1 Cut the white ends off the asparagus, then boil for 4–5 minutes or until tender.

2 Blend the asparagus in a blender or food processor with the crème fraîche, then place in a bowl. Add the remaining ingredients and stir to combine.

miso soup

MAKES **2 SERVINGS**

1 tablespoon red or white miso
½ small leek
50 g (2 oz) firm tofu
½ tablespoon wakame seaweed
chopped chives, to serve

Dashi stock:
8 g (¼ oz) kombu seaweed
900 ml (1½ pints) water
1 tablespoon dried tuna (bonito flakes) or
    1 tablespoon soy sauce

1 First make the dashi. Wipe the kombu seaweed with a damp cloth and place it in a saucepan with the water. Bring to a simmer, skimming away any scum that rises to the surface. When the soup is clear, add ½ tablespoon of the dried tuna flakes and simmer uncovered for 20 minutes. Remove the pan from the heat and add the remaining dried tuna flakes. Set aside for 5 minutes then strain the dashi and return to the pan.

2 Mix the miso with a little of the warm stock then add this a little at a time to the stock, stirring all the time until the miso has dissolved. Remove from the heat until ready to serve.

3 Cut the leek into fine julienne strips and the tofu into small squares. Warm the miso soup and add the leek and tofu with the wakame seaweed. Add the chives and serve immediately.

carrot and sage soup

MAKES **2 SERVINGS**

1 tablespoon olive oil
1 onion, finely chopped
375 g (12 oz) carrots, thinly sliced
450 ml (¾ pint) vegetable stock
1 tablespoon chopped sage leaves
salt and pepper
sage sprigs, to garnish (optional)

1 Heat the oil in a large heavy pan, add the onion and fry gently until soft but not golden, then add the carrots and stock. Season with salt and pepper. Bring to the boil and simmer, uncovered, for about 30 minutes.

2 Purée the soup in a food processor or blender until smooth, then return to the rinsed pan and add the chopped sage. Bring to the boil and simmer for another 15 minutes.

3 Serve the soup garnished with sage sprigs, if you like.

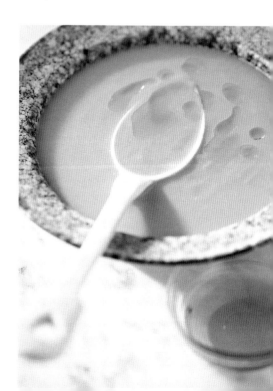

rice ball sushi
MAKES **2 SERVINGS**

125 g (4 oz) Japanese short-grain rice, rinsed
150 ml (¼ pint) cold water
½ teaspoon sugar
pinch of salt
1 tablespoon Japanese rice vinegar
25 g (1 oz) raw salmon, finely diced
wasabi paste, to taste
few slices of pickled ginger, plus extra to serve
1 teaspoon sesame seeds, toasted
½ sheet of nori seaweed
soy sauce, to serve

1 Put the rice in a heavy-based saucepan with the water. Cover the pan, bring to the boil and simmer for 20 minutes or until the rice is tender and the water absorbed. Remove from the heat, cover the pan with a tea towel and leave to stand for 10 minutes.

2 Put the sugar, salt and vinegar into a small saucepan and heat gently until the sugar has dissolved. Turn the rice out of the pan into a bowl and sprinkle with the vinegar. Toss gently with two forks to combine and to separate the rice grains as they cool.

3 Put a little of the rice in a damp egg cup and make a well in the centre. Add a little salmon, a smear of wasabi and a little pickled ginger. Press a little more rice over the top to seal. Shake the rice ball from the egg cup and mould into a ball with wet hands. Sprinkle with sesame seeds and repeat with the remaining rice and filling.

4 Toast the piece of nori lightly over a flame, then cut it into 2.5 cm (1 inch) strips with scissors. Wrap a strip of nori around each of the rice balls, sealing the ends together with a little water. Serve with soy sauce for dipping and pickled ginger.

chicken, avocado and mango salad
MAKES **1 SERVING**

bunch of watercress
2 cooked beetroots, sliced
½ avocado, sliced
½ mango, sliced
1 tablespoon lemon juice
125 g (4 oz) lean roast chicken, shredded
1 tablespoon chopped chives
1 tablespoon shredded basil leaves
pepper

1 Arrange the watercress and beetroot on a plate. Top with the avocado and mango slices, then sprinkle with a little lemon juice and season with pepper.

2 Place the chicken on top, sprinkle the chopped chives and shredded basil over the salad and serve.

salad niçoise
MAKES **1 SERVING**

50 g (2 oz) green beans
50 g (2 oz) asparagus
75 g (3 oz) new potatoes
handful of baby spinach leaves
1 chopped tomato
½ red onion, sliced
 splash of lemon juice
1 egg, boiled and sliced
50 g (2 oz) tuna in brine, drained or 25 g (1 oz) low-fat feta cheese, grated
pepper

1 Blanch the green beans and asparagus in boiling water until just tender, drain and refresh under cold running water and drain again. Boil the potatoes until tender.

2 Arrange the spinach, beans, asparagus and potatoes on a plate and top with the tomato and onion slices. Drizzle over a little lemon juice, then place the egg and tuna or cheese on top. Season well with pepper and serve.

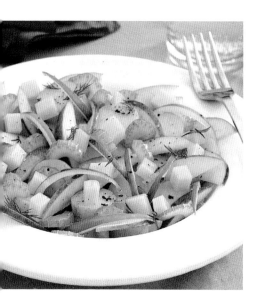

bean salad
MAKES **1 SERVING**

50 g (2 oz) canned kidney beans, rinsed and
   drained
75 g (3 oz) sliced green beans
25 g (1 oz) canned chickpeas, rinsed and drained
¼ onion, finely chopped
½ red pepper, finely chopped
1 teaspoon chopped coriander
1 teaspoon olive oil
pepper

Mix all the ingredients together in a bowl and
season with pepper.

watercress, mushroom and asparagus frittata
MAKES **2 SERVINGS**

6 asparagus stalks
4 eggs
½ bunch of watercress, tough stalks removed
1 small garlic clove, crushed
1 tablespoon olive oil
175 g (6 oz) mushrooms
pepper

1 Steam or boil the asparagus until just
tender, then refresh under cold running
water and drain well.

2 Beat the eggs in a bowl with a fork, then season
well with pepper and stir in the watercress.

3 Heat the oil in a heavy-based frying pan.
Add the mushrooms and garlic and fry
quickly for 3 minutes. Pour in the egg mixture
and arrange the asparagus evenly in the pan.

4 Reduce the heat to its lowest setting and
cook gently until the mixture is lightly set
and the underside is golden when the edge of
the frittata is lifted with a palette knife.

5 If the base of the frittata starts to burn
before the top is set, place the pan under a
moderate grill to finish cooking the top.

potato, celery and apple salad
MAKES **1 SERVING**

75 g (3 oz) new potatoes
1 crisp dessert apple, cored and sliced
1 tablespoon lemon juice
2 celery sticks, thinly sliced
50 g (2 oz) half-fat Cheddar cheese
¼ red onion, thinly sliced
½ tablespoon wine vinegar
1 tablespoon apple juice
½ teaspoon mild French mustard
1 tablespoon sunflower oil
pepper
dill or chervil sprigs, to garnish

1 Cook the potatoes in boiling water until
just tender. Drain and allow to cool, then
slice them carefully.

2 Sprinkle the apples with a little of the
lemon juice. Mix together the potatoes,
apples, celery, cheese and onion. In a small
bowl, beat together the remaining lemon juice,
vinegar, apple juice, mustard and oil. Season
with pepper to taste. Pour the dressing over
the potato mixture and mix thoroughly. Serve
garnished with dill or chervil sprigs.

braised lentils with mushrooms and gremolata

MAKES **2 SERVINGS**

2 tablespoons olive oil
1 onion, chopped
1 celery stick, sliced
1 carrot, sliced
75 g (3 oz) Puy lentils, rinsed
300 ml (1/2 pint) vegetable stock
125 ml (4 fl oz) dry white wine
1 bay leaf
1 tablespoon chopped thyme
175 g (6 oz) mushrooms, sliced
salt and pepper

gremolata:
1 tablespoon chopped parsley
finely grated rind of 1/2 lemon
1 garlic clove, chopped

1 Heat 1 tablespoon of the olive oil in a saucepan and fry the onion, celery and carrots for 3 minutes. Add the lentils, stock, wine, herbs, a generous seasoning of pepper and a small pinch of salt. Bring to the boil, reduce the heat and simmer gently, uncovered, for about 20 minutes, or until the lentils are tender.

2 Meanwhile, mix together the ingredients for the gremolata.

3 Heat the remaining oil in a frying pan, add the mushrooms and fry quickly for about 2 minutes until golden.

4 Ladle the lentils on to serving plates, top with the mushrooms and serve scattered with the gremolata.

aubergine towers

MAKES **2 SERVINGS**

2 small aubergines, about 12 cm (5 inches) long
1 tablespoon extra-virgin olive oil, plus extra for brushing
1/2 small onion, finely chopped
1 garlic clove, crushed
1 teaspoon grated lemon rind
1/2 teaspoon ground cumin
pinch of ground cinnamon
25 g (1 oz) sultanas
25 g (1 oz) cashew nuts, toasted and chopped
1 teaspoon tahini paste
25 g (1 oz) sun-dried tomatoes in oil, drained and chopped
1 tablespoon fresh coriander
salt and pepper

1 Cut off the stem of each aubergine about 2.5 cm (1 inch) from the top. Cut a slice from the bottom so that the aubergines will stand upright. Carefully scoop out the flesh, leaving the skin intact. Chop the flesh.

2 Heat the oil in a frying pan and fry the onion, garlic, lemon rind and spices for 5 minutes. Add the aubergine flesh and continue to cook for a further 6–8 minutes until tender. Stir in all the remaining ingredients and season to taste.

3 Spoon the filling mixture into the aubergines, brush with oil and arrange upright in a small roasting pan. Add about 1cm (1/2 inch) of boiling water and place in a preheated oven at 200°C (400°F), Gas Mark 6 for 40 minutes until cooked thoroughly. Serve immediately.

eggs benedict
MAKES **1 SERVING**

1 large flat-cap mushroom, stalk trimmed
1 tablespoon extra-virgin olive oil
125 g (4 oz) spinach, trimmed
pinch of nutmeg
1 small egg
25 g (1 oz) half-fat cheese
cayenne pepper

1 Place the mushroom, cap side down, in an ovenproof dish. Drizzle over the olive oil, cover with foil and place in a preheated oven at 200°C (400°F), Gas Mark 6 for 20 minutes.

2 Meanwhile, wash the spinach and place in a large saucepan. Heat gently until just wilted. Drain, squeeze out the excess liquid and chop roughly. Sprinkle with the nutmeg and stir to combine. Poach the egg in an egg poacher, or in a pan of gently simmering water, for 3–4 minutes until just cooked.

3 Remove the mushroom from the oven, spoon the chopped spinach around the mushroom and carefully place the poached egg on top. Sprinkle with the cheese and season with cayenne and place the dish under a preheated hot grill for 3–4 minutes until browned. Serve immediately.

lemon grass and tofu nuggets
MAKES **2 SERVINGS**

4 spring onions, roughly chopped
2.5 cm (1 inch) piece of fresh root ginger,
*   peeled and chopped*
1 lemon grass stalk, finely chopped
3 tablespoons chopped coriander
2 garlic cloves, roughly chopped
1/2 tablespoon light soy sauce
150 g (5 oz) tofu, drained
40 g (1 1/2 oz) breadcrumbs, made from
*   rye bread*
1/2 egg
1 tablespoon groundnut oil
pepper

1 Place the spring onions, ginger, lemon grass, coriander and garlic in a food processor and process lightly until mixed together and chopped, but still quite chunky. Add the soy sauce, tofu, breadcrumbs, egg and pepper and process until just combined.

2 Take dessertspoonfuls of the mixture and pat into flat cakes using wet hands. Place on a lightly greased grill pan and brush with a little oil. Grill under a preheated hot grill for 2–3 minutes on each side until golden. Serve immediately.

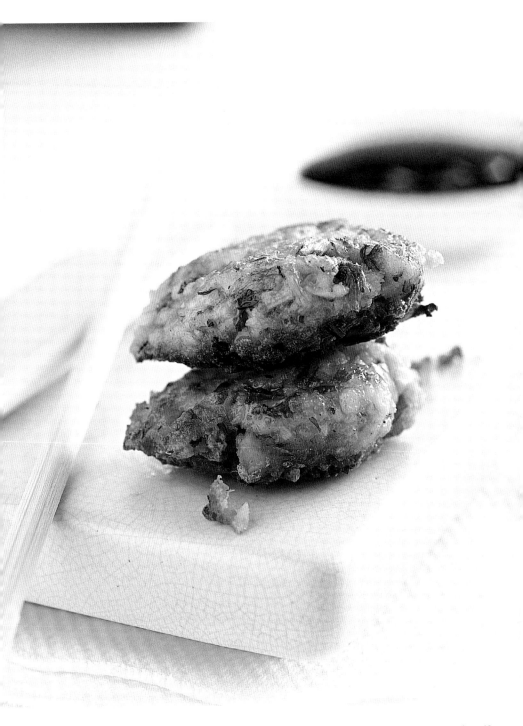

cabbage, beetroot and apple sauté
MAKES **2 SERVINGS**

1 tablespoon olive oil
1/4 red cabbage, thinly shredded
1/2 tablespoon chopped thyme
1 teaspoon caraway seeds
1/2 teaspoon ground mixed spice
1 teaspoon sugar
75 ml (3 fl oz) red wine
1 tablespoon port
1 tablespoon red wine vinegar
1 dessert apple, quartered, cored and
    thickly sliced
125 g (4 oz) cooked beetroot, cubed
125 g (4 oz) canned kidney beans, rinsed
    and drained
25 g (1 oz) pecan nuts, toasted
pepper

1 Heat half the olive oil in a large frying pan and fry the cabbage, thyme, caraway seeds, spice and sugar for 10 minutes. Add the wine, port and vinegar and bring to the boil. Cover the pan and cook over a low heat for 20 minutes.

2 Meanwhile, heat the remaining oil in a clean frying pan and fry the apples for 4–5 minutes until lightly golden. Add to the cabbage with the pan juices, the beetroot and the beans. Cover and cook for a further 15–20 minutes until the cabbage is tender. Season to taste with pepper. Stir in the nuts and serve at once.

mexican soup with avocado salsa
MAKES **2 SERVINGS**

1 tablespoon sunflower oil
1 onion, chopped
1 garlic clove, crushed
1 tablespoon ground coriander
1/2 teaspoon ground cumin
1/2 red pepper, cored, deseeded and diced
1 red chilli, deseeded and diced
200 g (7 oz) canned kidney beans, rinsed and drained
375 ml (13 fl oz) tomato juice
1/2–1 tablespoon chilli sauce (to taste)

avocado salsa:
1/2 small ripe avocado
2 spring onions, finely chopped
1/2 tablespoon lemon juice
1/2 tablespoon chopped fresh coriander
salt and pepper

1 Heat the oil in a large saucepan, add the onion, garlic, spices, pepper and chilli and fry gently for 10 minutes. Add all the remaining ingredients, bring to the boil and simmer gently for 30 minutes.

2 Meanwhile, make the avocado salsa. Peel, stone and finely dice the avocado and combine with the remaining ingredients. Season lightly to taste and cover.

3 Process all the soup ingredients in a blender or food processor. Return to a clean saucepan, season to taste and heat thoroughly. Serve with the salsa.

colourful kebabs
MAKES **1 SERVING**

8 raw tiger prawns, peeled and deveined,
    or 8 cubes of Quorn
1 yellow pepper, cut into cubes
1/2 onion, cut into chunks
4 mushrooms, halved
4 cherry tomatoes
1 teaspoon olive oil
1 teaspoon finely chopped rosemary or thyme
pepper

Thread the prawns or Quorn, pepper, onions, mushrooms and tomatoes on to 2 skewers. Brush with the oil and sprinkle with the herbs and pepper. Cook for 6–7 minutes under a preheated moderate grill until lightly charred. Serve at once.

poached salmon with hot basil sauce
MAKES **2 SERVINGS**

1 small bunch of basil
2 celery sticks, chopped
1/2 carrot, chopped
1/2 small courgette, chopped
1/2 small onion, chopped
2 salmon steaks, about 125 g (4 oz) each
40 ml (1 1/2 fl oz) dry white wine
50 ml (2 fl oz) water
1/2 teaspoon lemon juice
1 teaspoon low-fat spread
salt and pepper
lemon slices, to serve

1 Strip the leaves from half the basil and set aside. Spread all the chopped vegetables over the bottom of a large flameproof casserole dish with a lid, press the salmon steaks into the vegetables and cover them with the remaining basil, reserving a few leaves for garnishing. Pour over the wine and water and season lightly with salt and pepper. Bring to the boil, cover and simmer for about 10 minutes. Transfer the salmon to a warmed serving dish.

2 Bring the poaching liquid and vegetables back to the boil and simmer for 5 minutes. Strain into a food processor or blender and add the cooked and uncooked basil. Blend to a purée and return to a saucepan. Bring the purée to the boil and reduce by half, until thickened. Remove the saucepan from the heat, add the lemon juice and stir in the low-fat spread. Pour the sauce over the salmon steaks, garnish with the reserved basil leaves and serve with lemon slices.

anglo-indian curry
MAKES **2 SERVINGS**

1 tablespoon sunflower oil
1 large onion, sliced
1 garlic clove, chopped
1/2 cooking apple, peeled, cored and chopped
1cm (1/2 inch) piece of fresh root ginger, peeled and grated
1 tablespoon curry powder
250 ml (8 fl oz) vegetable stock
125 g (4 oz) potatoes, peeled and diced
125 g (4 oz) carrots, peeled and sliced
125 g (4 oz) pumpkin, peeled, deseeded and cubed
125 g (4 oz) broccoli florets
125 g (4 oz) runner beans, sliced
25 g (1 oz) sultanas
125 g (4 oz) cooked peeled prawns or Quorn pieces
1/2 tablespoon grated fresh coconut
salt and pepper

1 Heat the oil in a large pan. Add the onion, garlic, apple and ginger and fry gently for 5 minutes, stirring occasionally. Stir in the curry powder and fry gently for a further 3 minutes, stirring constantly.

2 Add the stock and bring to the boil, stirring constantly, until the sauce thickens slightly. Add salt and pepper to taste, then lower the heat and simmer for 2 minutes.

3 Add the potatoes and carrots. Cover the pan and simmer for 10 minutes.

4 Add the pumpkin, broccoli, beans, sultanas and Quorn, if using. Cover and simmer for 5–10 minutes or until the broccoli is just tender, but still crisp and not broken up. Stir in the prawns, if using, and heat through gently. Sprinkle with the coconut and serve hot.

chicken, squash and sweet potato tagine
MAKES **2 SERVINGS**

1 tablespoon olive oil
2 boneless, skinless chicken breasts
1 large onion, finely chopped
2 garlic cloves, crushed
1 cinnamon stick, broken in half
250 g (8 oz) sweet potatoes, cut into small
*   cubes*
250 g (8 oz) squash or pumpkin, cut into small
*   cubes*
3 tablespoons chopped mixed parsley and mint
150 ml (¼ pint) chicken stock
salt and pepper

to garnish:
flaked almonds
parsley sprigs
mint sprigs

1 Heat the oil in a large heavy casserole. Add the chicken and brown evenly. Remove and keep warm. Add the onions to the casserole and cook until soft and lightly browned, adding the garlic and cinnamon when the onions are nearly done.

2 Stir in the sweet potatoes and squash or pumpkin, then return the chicken to the pan, add half of the parsley and mint and pour in the stock. Cover tightly and simmer very gently for about 45 minutes until the chicken and vegetables are tender.

3 Season lightly with salt and pepper, then stir in the remaining parsley and mint. Scatter over the almonds and serve garnished with parsley and mint sprigs.

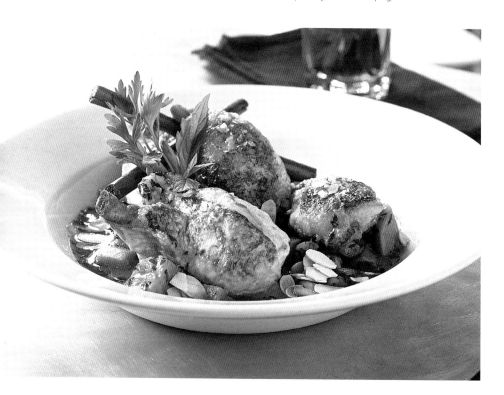

beef tacos

MAKES **2 SERVINGS**

250 g (8 oz) lean minced beef
40 g (1 1/2 oz) onion, finely chopped
50 g (2 oz) green pepper, cored, deseeded and
 finely chopped
1 garlic clove, crushed
1 teaspoon dried oregano
pinch of hot paprika
pinch of ground cumin
pinch of dried red hot-pepper flakes
50 ml (2 fl oz) tomato purée
6 corn taco shells
salt and pepper
paprika, to garnish

to serve:
shredded red cabbage
shredded red onion
grated carrot
1 tablespoon low-fat natural yogurt

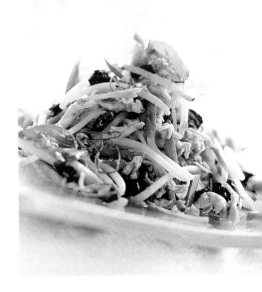

1 Put the minced beef in a frying pan and fry it gently in its own fat until it is cooked and browned, breaking it up as it cooks. Pour off and discard any excess fat. Add the onion, green pepper and garlic and cook, stirring occasionally, until softened. Stir in the oregano, spices and salt and pepper to taste, then add the tomato purée and mix well. Cover and cook gently for 10 minutes, stirring occasionally.

2 Meanwhile, heat the taco shells in a preheated oven at 180°C (350°F), Gas Mark 4. Serve the beef filling in the hot corn taco shells, accompanied by shredded red cabbage, onion and grated carrot. Drizzle with yogurt and sprinkle with paprika.

cranberry chicken stir-fry with ginger

MAKES **2 SERVINGS**

1 tablespoon vegetable oil
1 shallot, finely chopped
1 cm (1/2 inch) piece of fresh root ginger,
 chopped into matchsticks
1 garlic clove, crushed
2 boneless, skinless chicken breasts,
 thinly sliced
1 tablespoon hoisin sauce or dark soy sauce
1 tablespoon oyster sauce (optional)
1/2 tablespoon light soy sauce
15 g (1/2 oz) dried cranberries
2 spring onions, diagonally sliced
75 g (3 oz) bean sprouts, sliced peppers or
 carrot strips

1 Heat the oil in a wok and stir-fry the shallots, ginger and garlic for 30 seconds. Add the chicken and stir-fry for 2 minutes or until golden brown.

2 Add the hoisin, oyster and soy sauces and the cranberries and stir-fry for a further 2 minutes. Check that the chicken is cooked all the way through, then add the spring onions and bean sprouts or other vegetables and stir-fry for 4 minutes. Serve immediately.

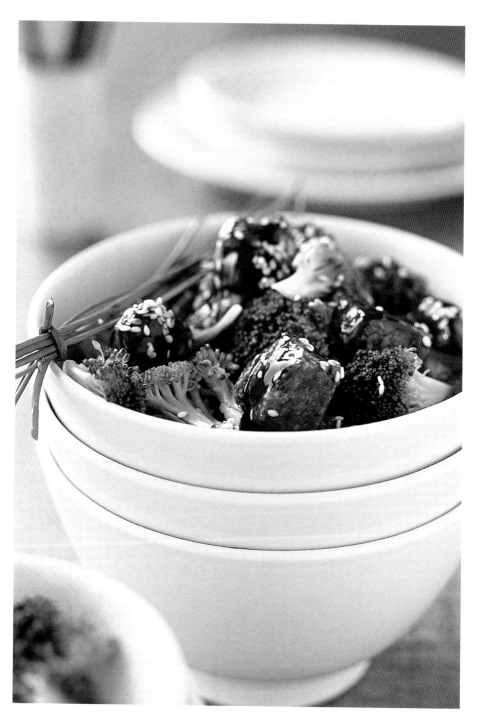

beef and broccoli with oyster sauce
MAKES **2 SERVINGS**

175 g (6 oz) rump steak, trimmed of all fat
1/2 egg white
1 tablespoon soy sauce
1 garlic clove, crushed
1 cm (1/2 inch) piece of fresh root ginger, grated
1/2 tablespoon cornflour
1 tablespoon groundnut oil
125 g (4 oz) broccoli, divided into small florets
50 ml (2 fl oz) Chinese rice wine or dry sherry
1 1/2 tablespoons oyster sauce
1 tablespoon soy sauce

to garnish:
1 tablespoon toasted sesame seeds
small bunch of chives, snipped (optional)

1 Wrap the beef in clingfilm and put it in the freezer for 1–2 hours until it is just hard.

2 Remove the beef from the freezer and unwrap it, then slice it into rectangles about the size of a large postage stamp, working against the grain. Whisk the egg white in a non-metallic dish, add the soy sauce, garlic, ginger and cornflour and whisk to mix. Add the beef, stir to coat, then leave to marinate at room temperature for about 30 minutes or until the beef is completely thawed out.

3 Heat the oil in a wok until very hot, but not smoking. Add half the beef rectangles and stir them around so they separate. Fry for 30–60 seconds until the beef changes colour all over, lift out with a slotted spoon and drain on kitchen paper. Repeat with the remaining beef.

4 Add the broccoli florets to the wok, sprinkle with the rice wine or sherry and toss over a moderate heat for 3 minutes. Return the beef to the wok and add the oyster sauce and soy sauce. Increase the heat to high and stir-fry vigorously for 3–4 minutes or until the beef and broccoli are tender. Serve hot, sprinkled with toasted sesame seeds. Garnish with snipped chives, if you wish.

hot thai beef salad
MAKES **2 SERVINGS**

1/2 crisp lettuce, shredded
40 g (1 1/2 oz) bean sprouts
1 ripe papaya, peeled and thinly sliced
1/4 large cucumber, cut into matchsticks
2 spring onions, cut into matchsticks
1 tablespoon vegetable oil
250 g (8 oz) rump or fillet steak, cut into thin
    strips across the grain
1 garlic clove, finely chopped
1 green chilli, thinly sliced
4 tablespoons lemon juice
1/2 tablespoon Thai fish sauce
1/2 teaspoon sugar

1 Place a pile of lettuce and bean sprouts on 2 individual plates and arrange the papaya, cucumber and spring onions to one side. Cover loosely and set aside.

2 Heat the oil in a heavy-based frying pan or wok over a moderate heat until hot. Add the beef, garlic and chilli, increase the heat to high and stir-fry for 3–4 minutes or until browned on all sides. Pour in the lemon juice and fish sauce, add the sugar and stir-fry until sizzling.

3 Remove the wok from the heat. Remove the beef from the dressing with a slotted spoon and divide between the two piles of lettuce and bean sprouts, arranging the papaya to one side and the cucumber and spring onions on top. Pour over the dressing and serve immediately.

sticking to the plan

We have already looked at some of the reasons why people fail to complete diet programmes (and hopefully proved that they shouldn't be a problem on this diet). However, there may be a few side effects that will affect you on the anti-cellulite programme, which could cause you to waver in your weight loss. These are cravings for some of the substances that are excluded from the plan. Here are some tips to help you get things back under control.

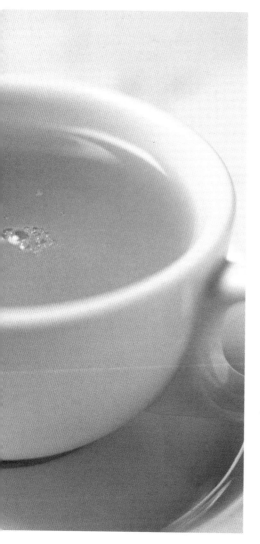

CAFFEINE

This is the most likely element of the Diet Solution to cause problems, as coming off caffeine can lead to headaches. There is also a psychological element to giving up caffeine: in one Harvard University trial, people who were told their coffee intake was being cut down suffered worse symptoms than those who were just given decaffeinated coffee on the sly. The good news is that you can drink coffee on the Diet Solution – but only up to three cups a day. If you are still suffering, try these ideas:

• Coffee substitutes such as chicory and barley, or teas like ginger and lemon, provide stimulation for body and mind – and satisfy the need to have a hot drink.

• The homoeopathic remedy coffea crudea (which is made from coffee beans) can help physical symptoms like headaches or jitters. It is available in health-food stores.

• Sprinkle 3–4 drops of lime, lemon or grapefruit essential oil on to a tissue and inhale to give you that energy boost.

• Try stimulating the acupressure point on your wrist to boost energy. Look for the crease closest to your palm and press the area directly below your thumb 5–10 times.

SUGAR

If you want to beat cellulite you have to cut down on sugar. The good news is that it takes just ten days for your tastebuds to become accustomed to life without sugar – after this you won't miss it. However, try the following tips to get you through those first few days:

- Take some rhodiola, a herb that can help balance your body against stress and fatigue. In trials it has been shown to increase levels of serotonin in the brain by 30 per cent and to balance blood sugar.

- Sniff some vanilla oil – studies at St George's Hospital in London have shown it reduces sugar cravings.

- Try gymnema sylvestre, a supplement that acts on the tastebuds so they can't detect sugar. The effects last about two hours, so use it when you know the cravings will be bad. Drink one cup of the tea or take one 100 mg supplement.

ALCOHOL

Many of us rely on a glass of wine or two to relax us in the evening. You are allowed one glass of wine or another alcoholic drink a night, but it will be easier to stick to this if you get your stress levels under control first. There are four simple fast fixes to lower your blood pressure if you feel yourself getting stressed:

- Warming your hands. When we are stressed, our temperature drops; by warming your hands you can raise your temperature and relax your system.

- Sniffing lavender oil. Conclusively proven to trigger calming alpha waves in the brain in a matter of minutes and known to reduce tension in muscles, lavender is the ultimate calmer.

- Deep breathing. Inhale for a count of 10, filling your abdomen, then your chest, then trying to expand your ribcage. Then exhale for a count of 20, deflating all those areas.

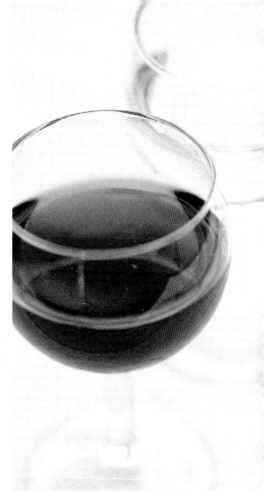

- If you still have problems, try the Chinese herb kudzu. In one UK trial, 64 per cent of volunteers said they were drinking less after taking the herb.

FAT

Many of us don't feel satisfied with a meal unless we have eaten some fat with it. The reason is that fat triggers our brains to feel happy and satiated after eating it. If you are really having trouble, finish each meal with a spoonful of low-fat crème fraîche, cottage cheese or natural yogurt, or a thin slice of edam or other low-fat cheese. The thick creamy texture can often trigger the sensation of fat.

eating out

The times when we are most vulnerable to giving up the eating plan are when we are eating out. This is often psychological – we think that because we are eating out, we should treat ourselves to whatever we want, and any 'normal' eating habits are forgotten.

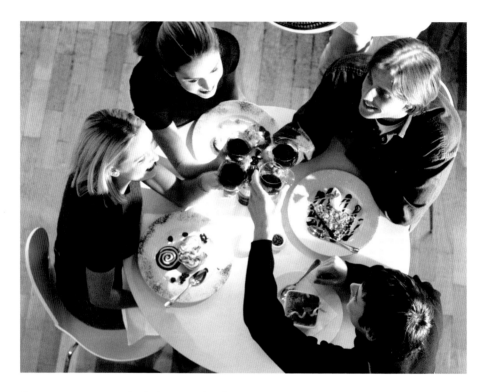

If you overeat once or twice in the six weeks of the programme, it won't matter. As long as you get straight back on the diet programme afterwards, you will still lose fat, fluid and your cellulite in six weeks.

However, if you eat out regularly, it could sabotage the anti-cellulite diet: big restaurant meals, sandwiches prepared at sandwich bars or fast-food fixes when you are eating on the run can all destroy that calorie limit in seconds and stop you seeing results. With that in mind, what follows is a list of meals that will fit into the anti-cellulite plan. Meals that you can

order with a (relatively) clear conscience if you are out and about.

Before you start ordering take-aways every night, though, remember this one study: researchers at the University of Memphis showed that women who ate out more than five times a week eat an average of 1,155 kJ (275 kcals) more per day – and 4 per cent more fat – than those who ate the same meals at home. This would cut your weight loss in half. Unless you are preparing food yourself, it is impossible to know just what is in the food and how many calories and grams of fat it contains.

ENERGY VALUES OF TYPICAL RESTAURANT FOOD

	kJ	kcal
English or American restaurant		
melon	420	100
tomato or mushroom soup	1,050	250
plain grilled steak without fat, with salad or vegetables	1,050	250
grilled or roast chicken without skin, with salad or vegetables	1,050	250
gammon steak with salad	1,890	450
grilled or seared fish or prawns, with salad or vegetables	1,470	350
plain jacket potato	840	200
Indian restaurant		
chicken tikka (starter portion)	1,050	250
tandoori chicken, one breast	1,470	350
plain prawn or chicken curry	1,470	350
vegetable curry	1,470	350
poppadum	315	75
boiled rice (per heaped tablespoon)	170	40
Chinese or Japanese restaurant		
chicken and sweetcorn, or hot and sour soup	630	150
beef/chicken in black bean or oyster sauce	1,470	350
stir-fried vegetables	1,050	250
steamed rice (per heaped tablespoon)	170	40
chop suey	1,260	300
sushi (per piece)	210	50
sashimi (per piece)	105	25
Italian restaurant		
minestrone soup	525	125
mozarella and tomato salad (starter portion)	1,155	275
parma ham with melon (starter portion)	630	150
seafood salad (starter portion)	1,050	250
veal dishes with side salad	1,470	350
pasta* with tomato or fish sauce	2,100	500

* Pasta is not on the anti-cellulite plan as it contains wheat. If you are eating Italian and don't eat meat, it may be unavoidable, so we have included it here. You may experience some fluid gain the day after you have eaten it, however.

	kJ	kcal
Fast-food restaurant		
six chicken nuggets or one breaded chicken piece	925	220
coleslaw (small portion)	500	120
main-course salads (beware creamy dressings and noodles, which can double that)	1,470	350
small portion of chilli	925	220
plain jacket potato	840	200
Sandwich bar		
jacket potato with baked beans, ratatouille, cottage cheese or coleslaw (without butter)	1,680 – 2,100	400–500
main-course salads (chicken, prawn, egg, tuna, no dressing)	1,470	350

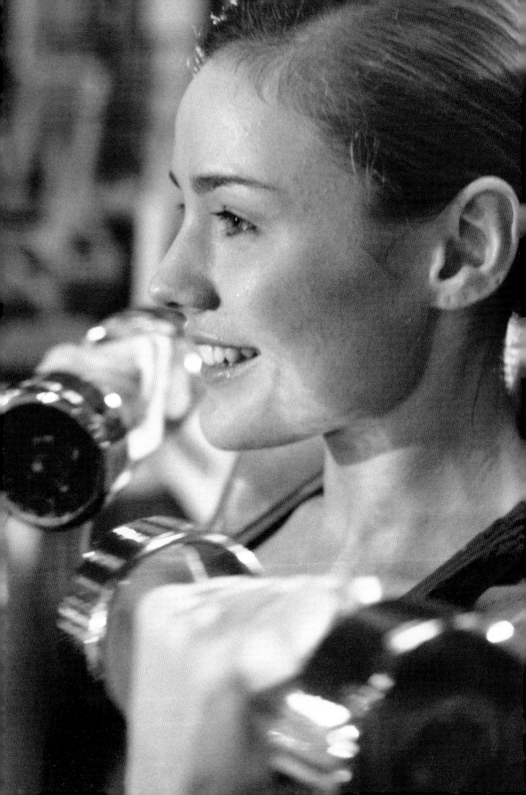

the
exercise solution

Exercise is one of the most effective ways to help reduce the look of lumpy thighs. A study at South Shore YMCA in Massachusetts put women on a relatively simple exercise programme for eight weeks. At the end of the study, 70 per cent said their cellulite had improved and on average they had lost 3.5 cm (1½ inches) from their hips. In another trial carried out by the University of Maryland, a number of women who were unhappy with the looks of their hips and thighs were put on a sensible diet and a programme of daily walking. At the end of the trial, they had a 4 per cent decrease in thigh circumference.

Exercise works on a number of levels. When you work out, you burn up to 15 times more calories than you do when you are sitting still. And even when you stop, your metabolic rate is increased, so you continue burning calories 6–10 per cent faster for up to 12 hours. This increases your ability to lose weight. You also lose weight because you gain muscle mass, and 0.5 kg (1 lb) of muscle burns 147 kJ (35 kcal) an hour, while fat burns none. Muscle also makes cellulite less noticeable as it stops the septa pulling down on the skin.

Exercise also stimulates the circulation. Five times more blood flows through your arteries and veins as you work out – and that blood is flooded with oxygen to feed the cells that form the septa.

In addition, exercise boosts the lymph flow. Unlike the circulation, the lymph system does not have a pump that propels it around the body. Instead it relies on the contraction of muscles to push it through the body – and as you exercise, the muscles contract. Put all this together and it's easy to see why exercise works so effectively to reduce cellulite. However, not all exercise works in the same way. For maximum benefit you need a combination of four distinctly different types of exercise tailored to your personal needs. In the Exercise Solution you'll learn exactly what these are, how to use them – and how to enjoy doing so.

CONTENTS

type 1: aerobic exercises

Aerobic exercise strengthens the heart and lungs, which means it can help fight cellulite by stimulating circulation and lymph flow. However, the main benefit is that it helps to burn calories and fat. If you are carrying excess weight (see page 15), this is the most important part of the Exercise Solution for you, so follow the fat-fighting plan below.

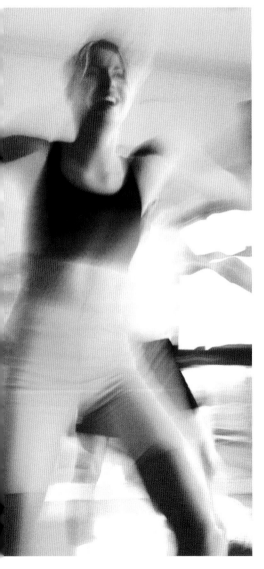

If you are not overweight, you will get most of your cosmetic benefits from the other exercises in the programme, though aerobic exercise will still benefit your health. You only need to do enough aerobic activity to give your circulation a regular burst. This means 30 minutes a day of climbing stairs, walking to the bus stop, gardening, disco dancing, or sports and formal exercise.

THE FAT-FIGHTING PLAN

You should already be losing 0.5 kg (1 lb) of fat per week on the Diet Solution, but you can increase this through exercise. Aim to burn 6,300–14,700 kJ (1,500–3,500 kcal) per week, in 3–5 sessions of working out. Your energy and fitness levels will dictate how much you can achieve – start off aiming for 6,300 kJ (1,500 kcal), then work up. Opposite you will see a box that tells you roughly how many calories you can burn in 30 minutes of some popular aerobic exercises. By mixing and matching these you can create your own work-out plan.

However, there is also a simple circuit-training plan overleaf. Circuit training is great for burning fat as it keeps your body moving, but because you swap from move to move you also stop boredom setting in. The routine is for 20 minutes (plus a five minute warm-up) and will burn roughly 1,050 kJ (250 kcal) when carried out by a 70 kg (11 stone) woman. Do this three times a week, plus a daily fast walk of 20 minutes, and you will be burning over 6,300 kJ (1,500 kcal) a week.

Never underestimate the little calorie burns you can work into your day. The average person climbing just two extra flights of stairs a day would burn enough calories over a year to lose 1.4 kg (3 lb). Think about how you can build activity into your day – getting off the bus a stop earlier, walking up (or even down) stairs, going round the block before you reach the sandwich bar, walking to accounts rather than emailing them, or you could try having a walk break instead of a coffee break.

Even pacing when you are on the phone will make a difference. The average office worker gets 48 phone calls a day. Even if each call lasts only a minute, if you walk backwards and forwards while you take them, you will do the equivalent of a 2.4 km (1½ mile) walk every day and can burn off 0.5kg (1 lb) of fat a month.

A good way to measure these extra bits of activity is to buy a pedometer and aim for 10,000 steps daily, the equivalent of a 8 km (5 mile) walk.

MIX-AND-MATCH EXERCISES

This table shows the calories burnt by a woman in 30 minutes of normal exercise (to convert to kilojoules, multiply by 4.2).

your weight	57 kg (9 stone)	63.5 kg (10 stone)	70 kg (11 stone)	76 kg (12 stone)
Aerobics (low-impact)	166	185	203	222
Aerobics (high-impact)	212	235	259	282
Step class (hard)	302	336	370	403
Water aerobics	121	134	148	161
Exercise bike (moderate)	212	235	259	282
Exercise bike (fast)	318	353	388	403
Rowing machine (moderate)	212	235	259	282
Stepper (moderate)	181	202	222	242
Cycling (outside)	242	269	296	323
Golf (carrying your clubs)	166	185	203	222
Hiking	181	202	222	242
Horse riding	121	134	148	161
Ice- or rollerskating	212	235	259	282
Skipping	300	336	370	403
Squash	210	235	259	282
Jogging (10 kph/6 mph)	300	336	370	403
Swimming	180	202	222	242
Tennis	210	235	259	282
Walking (6.5 kph/4 mph)	135	151	166	181

the circuit

Start with the warm-up, then follow this 20-minute programme in the order shown below, repeating the exercises from rope jumps four times. After you have finished, carry out the stretch programme shown opposite and overleaf.

As a general rule, with all the circuit exercises, you should aim to be working at 60–80 per cent of your maximum heart rate – this feels like you are working at about 7–8 on a scale, with 10 being the maximum you could manage. You should be able to speak while you are exercising, but not for more than five or six words.

warm-up (5 minutes)	Start by walking on the spot slowly for 1 minute, then increase your speed to a fast on-the-spot walk for another minute. For the last 3 minutes, work up to jogging on the spot, trying to go as fast as possible for the last minute.
rope jumps (1 minute)	Skip with a rope as fast as you can for a minute.
sprints (1 minute)	Run as fast as possible from one end of your garden – or sitting room – and back, first making sure nothing is in your way. If you find it hard to keep an intensive effort throughout, sprint out and jog more slowly back, gradually building up to full sprints as the weeks go on.
steps (1 minute)	Step up with one foot, then the other, on to the first step of a flight of stairs. Step back down with one foot, then the other. Repeat as fast as you can, but try to keep a strong steady rhythm. Be careful that when you step forward you don't push your knee too far in front.
star jumps (1 minute)	Jump up as fast as possible, and as you do, widen your legs and then your arms. Repeat, bringing your arms and legs back to the starting position. Repeat as many times as possible. To soften the impact on your knees and back, try to bend your knees slightly as you land and before you spring up.
jog on the spot (1 minute)	Aim to jog fast for a whole minute. If your fitness is limited, it is more important to keep up a steady pace for the whole minute than to go all out for 30 seconds and then have to stop. Start slow and work up to what feels comfortable.

stretches

At the end of any aerobic or toning exercises, you should stretch your muscles to reduce the risk of soreness or injury the next day. Here is a simple stretch routine.

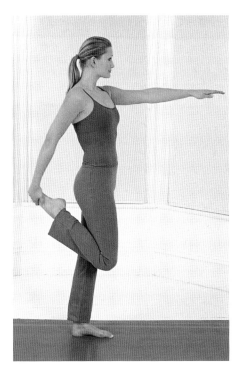

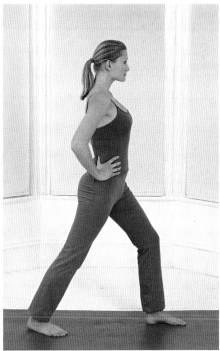

▲ 1 thigh stretch

- Stand up straight, then lift your right ankle up behind you, bending your knee. Grasp your foot and gently pull it towards your bottom. You will feel this stretch in your thigh.

- Hold for 30 seconds, putting out your other arm for balance if you need to.

- Lower the foot, then repeat with the other leg.

▲ 2 hamstring stretch

- Stand up straight, then straighten your right leg out, toe on the floor.

- Keeping this straight (but without locking your knees), gently bend the left leg and push the buttocks back as if you were going to sit down. You should feel this pull along the back of your thigh. Hold for 20–30 seconds, release and swap legs.

- Avoid this stretch if you have back problems.

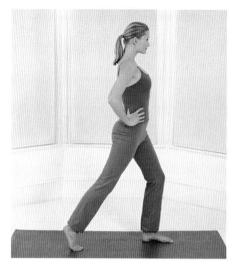

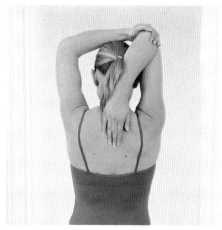

▲ 4 tricep stretch

- Reach your right hand up and over your shoulder so that your arm is bent with the elbow pointing upwards and the palm of your hand flat on your back.

- Using the other arm, gently press the upper arm backwards. Hold for 30 seconds, then swap sides.

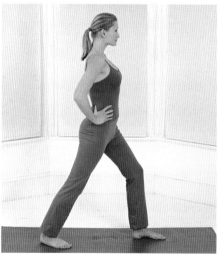

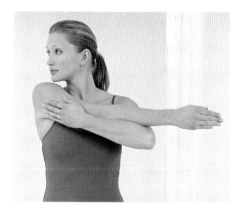

▲ 3 calf stretch

- Step forwards with your left leg and bend your knee. As you do this, your right leg will straighten and your right heel will come off the floor.

- Keeping your right leg straight, gently try to push your right heel back down. Hold for 30 seconds when you feel the stretch. Release gently and swap legs.

▲ 5 deltoid stretch

- Stand up straight and reach your right arm across your body at roughly shoulder height. Use your left arm placed just above the elbow to gently push your right arm closer to your body.

- Hold for 30 seconds, release, then swap arms.

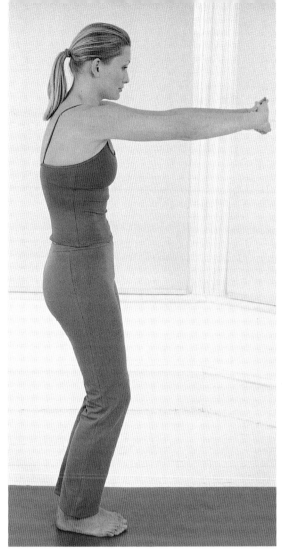

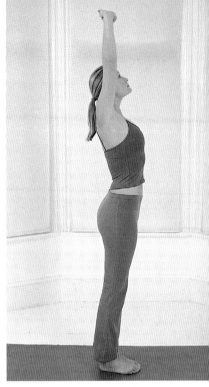

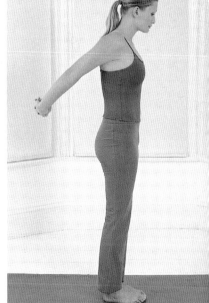

▲ 6 chest and shoulder stretch

• Link your fingers and, turning your palms outwards, push your hands forwards so you feel a stretch across your back and shoulders. Hold for 30 seconds, then release.

• Now push your arms up above your head so you feel the stretch up your torso and back. Hold for 30 seconds.

• Release, reach behind you and, again, link fingers. Gently pull your linked arms up until you feel the pull across your chest. Hold for 30 seconds, then release.

type 2: toning exercises

If you are slim, the toning programme will be very important to you. Apart from storing excess fluid, the main reason slim women develop cellulite is that they have poor muscle tone. The less muscle you have in your hips and thighs, the more the septa pull down against the skin and the more lumps and bumps are revealed. In addition to hiding the cellulite, muscle burns calories even while you are sitting still, so by toning up you will increase your metabolic rate and boost your weight-loss efforts – as well as creating tighter, tauter skin.

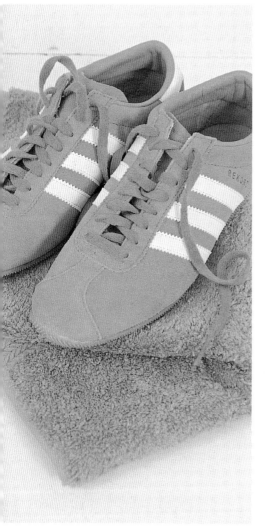

Everyone on the Exercise Solution needs to carry out the following 20-minute toning programme 3–5 times a week on alternate days. This spacing is really important: muscle is not built when you train, it is built on the days you rest. Don't worry that these exercises use weights – you will not develop huge muscles by doing these moves. You can do the exercises without dumb-bells, but you won't get the same results.

There are arm, shoulder and back exercises here – don't skip them thinking it's only your hips and thighs you want to change. The more muscle you have in your body, the more calories you burn, and a toned upper body can balance out a bottom-heavy figure. Finally, if you can't find 20 minutes every other day, don't panic. You can break up the toning exercises into tiny chunks – even just do one at a time – so long as they are all done during your 'toning day'.

WARM-UP
Spend 10 minutes walking, jogging, skipping, dancing or bouncing on a mini trampoline to warm up the body. You don't need to do this if you have just completed your aerobic work-out.

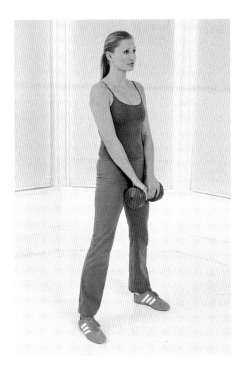

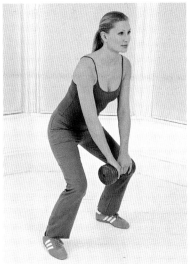

▲ 1 squats

- Stand up straight with feet hip-width apart. With arms straight, hold a 4–7 kg (9–15 lb) dumb-bell down between your legs.

- Keeping your arms as they are (they move with you), squat down as if you were going to sit in a chair. Make sure that you do this with your bottom muscles, not by widening your legs; your knees mustn't go further forwards than your ankles.

- Now use your thigh and buttock muscles to push yourself back up to a standing position. When you reach the top, clench your bottom and hold for one second; repeat 12 times. Then repeat the whole sequence four times.

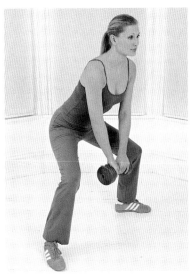

▲ 2 wide squats

- Stand in the same position as before.

- This time, take your legs wider apart and turn your feet out at 45 degrees. Perform exactly the same movement as before, watching your knees again.

- Again, do four sets of 12 repetitions.

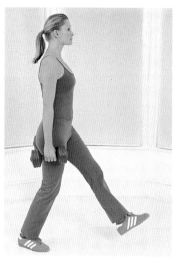
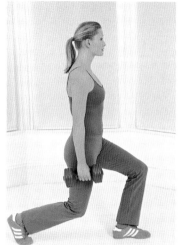

▲ 3 lunges

- Hold a dumb-bell in each hand, resting your arms by your sides.

- Now take a step forwards with your left leg and dip down, so your right knee bends towards the floor and your body goes with it. Make sure your knee doesn't go further forwards than your ankle and that your feet don't turn.

- Push up from your right foot (you should feel it in your bottom and inner thigh) and come back to a standing position. Do 12 movements, then repeat on the other leg.

- Now, repeat the whole thing four times.

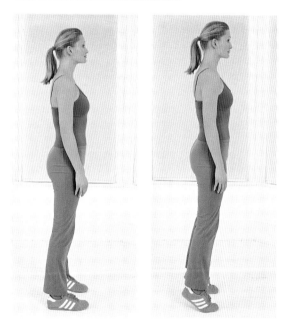

▲ 4 calf raises

- Stand up straight with your feet flat on the floor, but turned in so your toes are pointing slightly towards each other.

- Raise up on to your toes, tensing your calf muscle. Slowly lower back down. Repeat four sets of 12 repetitions.

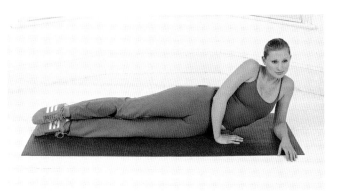

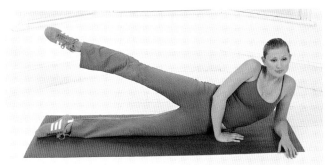

◀ 5 abductors

- Lie on your side with hips straight, legs one on top of the other.

- Slowly raise the top leg up and, when you reach as far as you can go, slowly pulse the muscle 30 times by pushing it out that little bit further.

- Relax. Switch legs and repeat. Work both legs three times each.

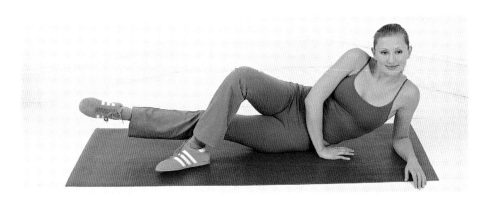

▲ 6 adductors

- Lie on your side with hips straight and legs outstretched. Bend the knee of the top leg and place your foot in front of the lower leg, so your foot is at 90 degrees to your lower leg.

- Now slowly lift the lower leg 5–7.5 cm (2–3 inches) off the floor. Lower. Repeat three sets of 20 repetitions.

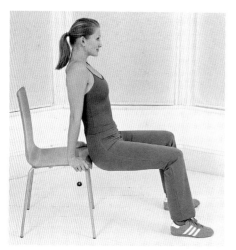 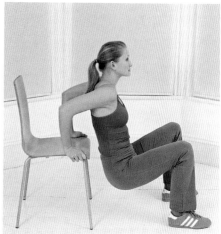

▲ 7 tricep dips

• Sitting on a sturdy chair, place your hands either side of your hips and grasp the edges of it. Keeping your body straight, lower yourself off the chair. Use your arms to raise and lower your body up and down by about 15 cm (6 inches), keeping your hips close to the chair.

• Work up to four sets of 12 repetitions.

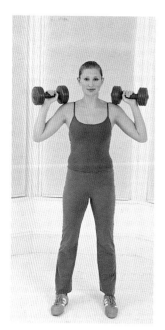 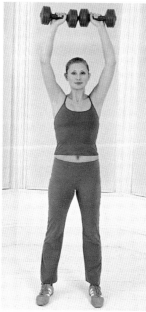

◀ 8 shoulder raises

• Stand up straight with a 2–5 kg (4½–11 lb) dumb-bell in each hand.

• Raise your arms up to shoulder height, then bend at the elbows so your palms are in the air. Raising from the shoulders, straighten your arms to just before your elbows lock and bring the dumb-bells together.

• You should feel this across your back and shoulders. Repeat four sets of 12 repetitions.

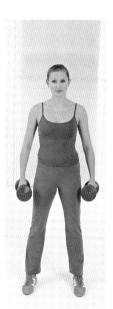
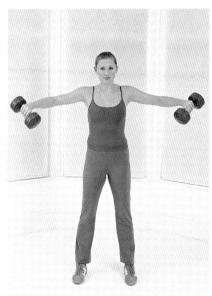

◀ 9 dumb-bell flies

- Stand up straight, arms by your sides, elbows bent and holding a dumb-bell in each hand. Lifting from your shoulders, raise your arms so your upper arms are parallel with your shoulders.

- Slowly lower and repeat four sets of 12 repetitions.

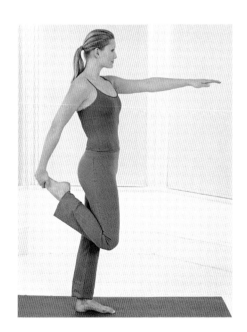

▲ 10 stretch routine

- Carry out the stretch routine on page 65.

IN THE GYM

If you belong to a gym, you can replace this programme by using the weights machines. Carry out the following circuit 3–5 times a week. For each exercise, work at a weight that means the last one of each repeat feels almost impossible to carry out.

warm-up	As above
leg press	3 sets of 12 repetitions
leg curl	3 sets of 12 repetitions
abductor	3 sets of 12 repetitions
adductor	3 sets of 12 repetitions
lunges	As above
calf raises	As above
lateral pulldowns	3 sets of 12 repetitions
shoulder press	3 sets of 12 repetitions
chest press	3 sets of 12 repetitions
stretch	As above

type 3: lymph-boosting exercises

These are important exercises for anyone for whom fluid storage causes cellulite. They aim to stimulate the lymph and get it flowing, reducing the amount of fluid the cellulite cells retain (see page 13). While all exercise will help to do this, the following 10-minute programme is tailored specifically towards stimulating lymph flow. It uses yoga moves that aim directly to stimulate the lymph and move its flow towards the main excretion points – the armpits and groin. When you do these exercises, you help cleanse the lymph faster, preventing toxic overload.

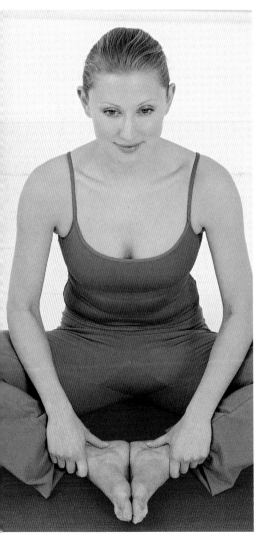

Everyone on the Exercise Solution should carry out the lymph-boosting programme at least three times a week. However, if you really do have problems with fluid retention, aim for 5–7 sessions a week. It takes only about 10 minutes and, as it is energizing, is a great thing to do just before breakfast.

◀ 1 yoga breathing

This starts the programme by filling the lungs with clean air and energizing your system ready for what follows.

- Lie on your back with your legs straight, and press your lower back into the floor. If you find this hard, bend your knees instead.

- Put your fingers on your naval, and breathe in and out a few times.

- Now, this time when you inhale, aim to fill your lungs from the bottom so that your tummy balloons out, then fill the middle of the lungs and finally the chest. Aim to breathe in for a count of five.

- Now exhale for a count of ten, letting the air out of the belly first, then the middle and finally the top of the lungs.

- Repeat five times.

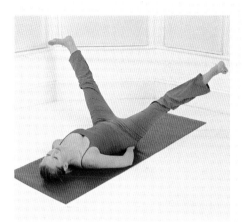

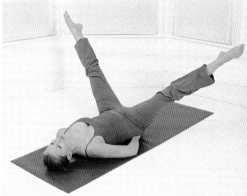

▲ 2 leg vibrations

This exercise helps stimulate the blood flow in the legs.

- Lie on your back and put your legs in the air. Open them and very slowly rotate your ankles to the left five times, then the right.

- Now stretch your toes to the ceiling and hold them there for a count of five.

- Bend your feet halfway back to their normal position and hold for five.

- Now push the feet towards your shins and hold for five.

- Put your feet back into their natural position, then tense your legs and try to find a point at which they naturally start to vibrate. This sounds strange, but it will happen. This gentle vibration dramatically stimulates blood flow to the groin. Let yourself 'wobble' for up to two minutes.

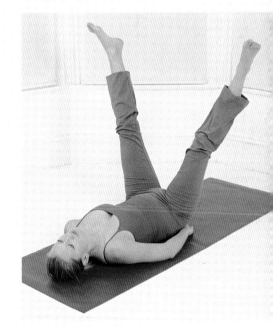

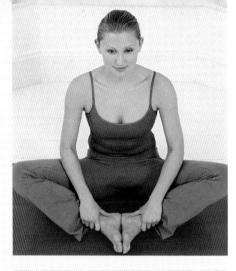

4 cat and dog tilts

These poses stimulate the kidneys and colon, helping to remove toxins from the system.

- Kneel on all fours. Keep your elbows locked and your neck straight.

- Now inhale and, as you do, push your body down and forwards to gently arch your back and straighten your arms. Lead with your chin as if you are trying to dip under a rope.

- Exhale and, as you do this, round your back so your head drops between your hands. Keep your tummy and buttocks tight.

- Repeat the whole sequence four times.

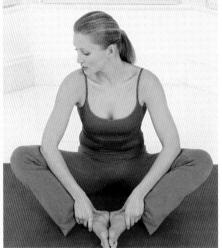

▲ 3 butterfly

This pose stimulates the blood flow around the hips.

- Sit on the floor with legs apart, but with knees bent and the soles of your feet together, back straight.

- Rest hands on ankles with arms by your sides.

- Exhale and, as you do this, bring your knees upwards so they press against your arms.

- Inhale and press them back down.

- Repeat ten times.

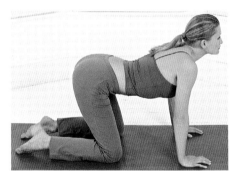

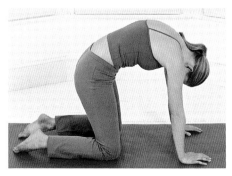

▷ 5 skytower

This stimulates lymph throughout the upper body.

- Stand up straight with feet together, your buttocks and tummy tucked in and tight. Place your arms by your sides.

- Inhale and, as you do, turn your palms outwards, then raise your arms slowly out to shoulder height, then above your head.

- Clench your palms together, pointing your index fingers to the sky, and stretch upwards throughout your whole body. Hold for 5 seconds.

- Exhale and go back to the start. Repeat five times.

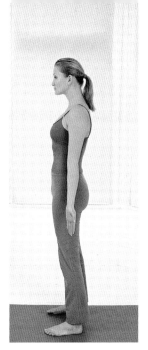
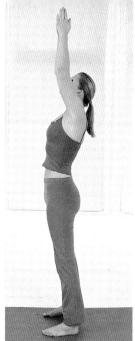

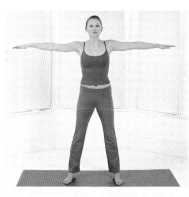
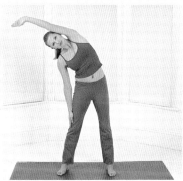

◁ 6 fishhook

This stimulates the blood flow and lymph in the armpits, a major point of elimination for the body.

- Stand with your legs apart and your feet pointing straight ahead.

- Breathe in, stretch out your arms and raise them to shoulder height.

- Exhale slowly and, as you do, drop your right arm to your side.

- Inhale and lift your left arm up alongside your head (close to your ear), twisting it so your palm faces the sky. Keep your hips facing forwards and bend gently sideways.

- Hold for 5–10 seconds, exhale slowly, then return to the start point.

- Repeat on the other side.

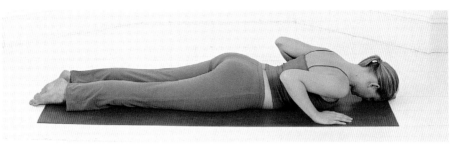

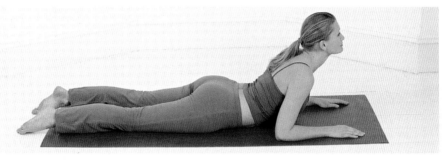

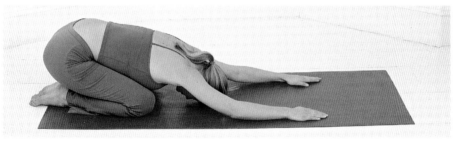

▲ 7 the cobra

This final exercise is the ultimate detox move and aims to move any unprocessed toxins to the kidneys, liver and bowel.

- Lie on your front with your head on the floor and your hands under your shoulders. Your heels should be together and your buttocks clenched.

- Exhale and roll your head gently off the floor.

- Inhale and lift your head, shoulders and chest off the floor. For a further stretch, continue this ╌e by straightening your arms; otherwise keep bent.

- Exhale and lower back down. When you reach your start position, gently push your buttocks back so that you feel a stretch along your back and end up sitting on your heels. Relax in this position for a few seconds.

- Repeat the exercise three times. The last time, relax for a little longer and slowly rise up on to your heels, progressing to a standing position. Your head should remain bowed as you do this and only be brought up when you are completely erect.

- Spend one minute carrying out the yoga breathing from step 1 (see page 74) and you're done.

type 4: posture exercises

Having poor posture is like putting bends in a straight road. Lymph and other fluids that used to flow smoothly get slowed up in certain areas. The result is congested muscles and tissues in the back and surrounding areas that can then reduce lymph flow throughout the whole system.

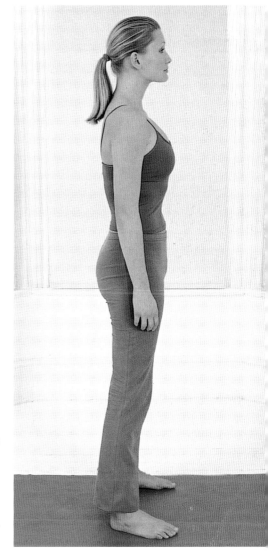

Poor posture also reduces the efficacy of breathing, reducing circulation and decreasing the elimination of natural toxins like carbon dioxide, which puts pressure on the lymph system. If you do suffer from any of the above problems, the following exercises can help by straightening posture, releasing tension and strengthening the core muscles that support the back.

▶ 1 to stand correctly

- The easiest way to ensure you are standing in the best position is to focus on lengthening your torso and tightening your tummy muscles. As you do this, everything else adjusts.

- Stand up, then focus on pulling and lengthening your body up, starting at your neck and pulling up through your chest to your waist and hips. Imagine a string pulling you upwards, and that the gap between your ears and your shoulders is lengthening, that each vertebra is spreading out from its neighbours and that your knees and ankles are lengthening and pulling out.

- Once you've done this, focus on pulling your tummy muscles back towards your navel – this doesn't mean holding your breath or squishing in your tummy. Instead, just contract the area around your navel so it feels as if your belly button is pushing towards your back. This supports your body. It may feel hard at first, but try to keep it up. A good way to remember is to place sticky red dots on your computer or around your home. Every time you see the dots, focus on putting your body in the right position and eventually it will come naturally.

▶ 2 to release tension

Poor posture can be aggravated by holding your body in the same position for hours each day, as you do when you are working at a computer. Once every hour, try this set of desk exercises.

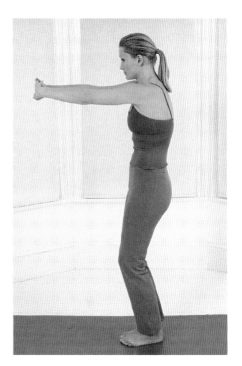

- Sitting straight, shrug your shoulders up towards your ears. As you go up, tense all the muscles, then release on the way down. Repeat 4–5 times.

- Interlock your fingers and, turning your palms to face outwards, straighten your arms out in front of you. Push gently forwards so you feel the stretch along your shoulder blades. Hold for 10 seconds.

- Keeping your fingers interlocked, push your arms up above your head and stretch your torso upwards. Hold for 10 seconds.

- Finally, tip your head gently to one side so you feel a stretch on the side of your neck. Hold for 10 seconds. Bring your head back to the centre, then tip to the other side and hold.

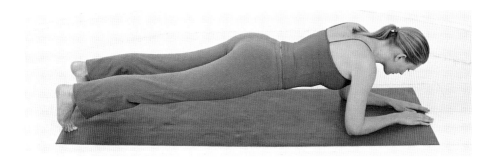

▲ 3 to strengthen the core muscles

Core muscles are those within the abdomen that stabilize the back and help improve posture. These exercises work alongside the upper body exercises in the toning plan to create a strong and healthy support for your whole body. Do them every two days throughout the programme – perhaps at the end of your toning regime.

- Get into a press-up position, but instead of balancing on your hands, balance on your elbows with your palms on the floor. Make sure your back is flat. Now pull in your stomach (not by breathing, but by pulling in the muscles) to create a dead-straight line with your body. Be careful not to arch your back as you do this. Hold for 15 seconds without holding your breath. Repeat up to five times.

▶ 4 raises

- Get down on all fours. Now try to raise your right arm and your left leg and hold for 30 seconds. As you do this, focus on using your core muscles to keep you stable. That is what is important, not the leg or arm movement. Hold for 15 seconds, then repeat five times. Switch so that you raise your right arm and left leg and repeat.

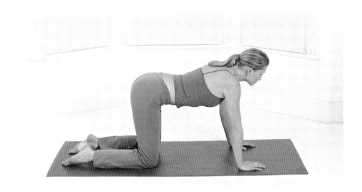

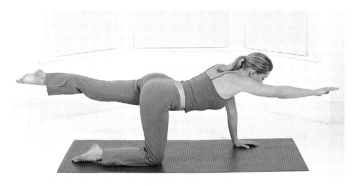

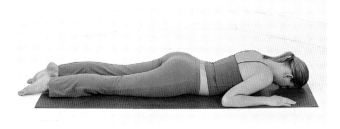

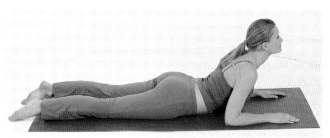

◀ 5 lower back curl

- Lie on the floor, elbows and forearms resting on the ground, palms just ahead of your ears. Slowly and gently raise up on to your forearms, arching your back from the waist. Hold for 2–3 seconds and slowly lower. Repeat ten times.

motivation tips

There is, unfortunately, rather a lot of exercise in the cellulite Solutions programme and you may find it difficult if you don't enjoy exercise. If you are finding it hard to get started, or if you are halfway through the programme and find that you are losing interest, you need to give your motivation a kick-start. Here are some tips that will help.

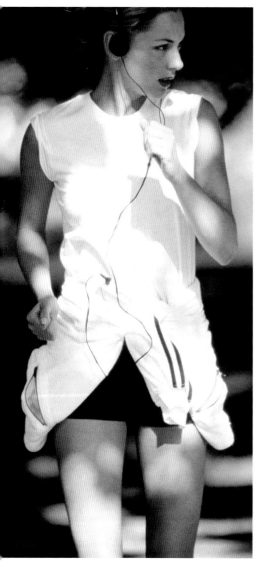

DON'T FOCUS ON WEIGHT LOSS OR A VISIBLE REDUCTION IN YOUR CELLULITE

While these are the ultimate goals, focusing on them will not motivate you to exercise, as changes are slow and steady. Instead, create an exercise-related goal for yourself. Try to do more star jumps in a minute every session, or run a little further in 20 minutes than you did last week. If, every time you work out, you set yourself an achievable goal to beat, you'll work harder and get more satisfaction (when you beat it) than you would just by heading out. If you don't like competing with yourself, set fun challenges instead – try to climb the Empire State Building (1,860 steps) over a week on a step machine or by going up and down the stairs at home.

DON'T DO THE SAME WORKOUT MORE THAN THREE DAYS IN A ROW

Variety is the key to preventing boredom in every area of your life and exercise is no exception. Every couple of sessions, change something about your workout – do things in a different order or run a different route; try a different sport or just do the one you normally do faster or more intensely. Not only does this keep your mind occupied, it also keeps your muscles stimulated and increases results.

USE EXTERNAL MOTIVATORS

Studies have shown that people who work out to music exercise 25 per cent longer than those who don't keep to the beat. Home workers who exercised in front of the television stayed put longer than normal. Research has even found that cyclists who sniffed citrus scents before they started found their workout easier than it actually was – and they enjoyed it more. Think what will keep you exercising and use it.

WORK OUT WITH A FRIEND

Indiana University scientists found that people who exercised with a friend were seven times more likely to stick to their programme than those working out solo. Just never arrange to meet your partner at the gym or swimming pool itself – you are more likely to turn up if you think of them standing on a street corner.

TRY THE 10-MINUTE RULE

If you don't think you want to exercise, tell yourself you will do 10 minutes and then see how you feel. If you are still not in the mood when you reach that point, you can stop. However, if your mood changes and you feel up to it, you will carry on. Nine times out of ten you

will carry on. The day you don't is a day you really did need to take a break – don't beat yourself up about it. Rest days are essential to every exerciser sometimes – just try not to go more than 72 hours without a workout. The endorphins (happy hormones) produced when you work out hang around for 72 hours, making your next workout in this time feel easier. If you wait longer, it is like starting from scratch and you are more likely to feel like quitting.

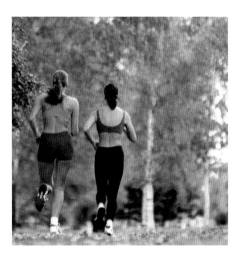

WHAT TO DO WHEN

Here is your at-a-glance guide to exactly what types of exercise you should be doing when.

exercise type	if you are trying to burn fat	if you are not trying to burn fat
aerobic	3–5 times a week, aiming to burn at least 6,300 kJ (1,500 calories)	3 times a week for 20 minutes
toning	3–5 times a week for 20 minutes – on alternate days	3–5 times a week for 20 minutes – on alternate days
lymph-boosting	3–7 times a week	3–7 times a week
posture	3–5 times a week	3–5 times a week

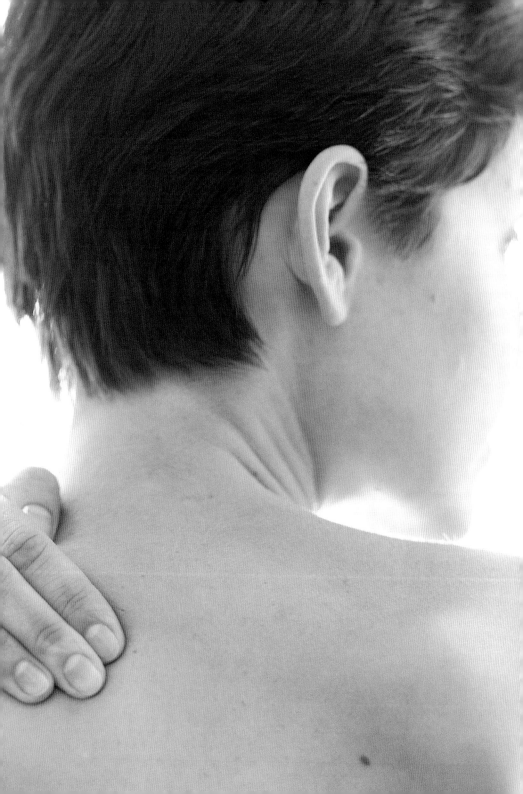

the stimulating solution

As we have already seen, poor circulation and lymph flow play a major part in the formation of cellulite. Just to remind you why, poor circulation deprives the body of oxygen – when this happens, the fibroblast cells that mend damaged collagen act abnormally, creating thick fibres that make fat stores more likely to bulge from the tops of their 'boxes'. On top of this, a sluggish lymph system increases the risk of water retention and also adds to the thicker collagen fibres with fibres of its own.

Boosting lymph and circulation is therefore a vital part of fighting cellulite and, by following the tips in the Stimulating Solution, you aim to do just this. What's more, by stimulating the circulation you could even improve the chance of the Diet Solution taking the weight from your hips and thighs rather than focusing primarily on your upper body. This is because when the body doesn't have enough sugar in the blood or muscles to use as energy, it reaches into the fat stores for fuel – and the stores it reaches first are those with the best circulation. By stimulating circulation and blood flow in your hips and thighs, you increase the chance that fat will be taken from there.

There are a number of ways you can stimulate circulation, but the Stimulating Solution focuses on skin brushing, massage, and heat and water treatments. These are treatments commonly used in health spas and beauty centres to help clients fight cellulite, and there is a scientific basis behind them. Chinese researchers have proven that during massage, gaps open up between cells and speed up lymph flow; and research looking into the use of hot spas has found that not only do these boost circulation, they may even aid weight loss. But despite their professional reputation, these techniques are safe and simple enough to be carried out at home – and take a matter of minutes to carry out. In many cases it will take just 10 minutes a day to get results.

CONTENTS

skin brushing

Skin brushing is the most commonly prescribed treatment for cellulite and one of the easiest to use. It uses gentle upwards movements to help boost circulation and lymph flow.

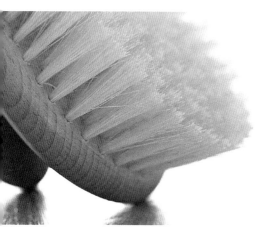

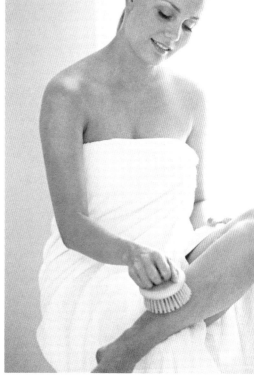

Skin brushing is best carried out in the morning before you bath or shower (while the skin is dry). As well as improving circulation, it also helps to get rid of dead skin cells that can lead to dry, dehydrated skin, under which cellulite is far more noticeable. Although you may be tempted to concentrate on cellulite areas alone, a complete body brush will ensure that your overall circulation is improved and will stimulate major lymph areas, including those under the arms and in the neck.

Choose a natural bristle brush with medium-hard bristles. Synthetic bristles or those that are too hard can scratch the skin. The head of the brush should be about the size of your hand, with a short or medium handle to reach hard places. Wash your brush once a week with a little shampoo and hang it up to dry. Mould can easily grow on dirty or damp brushes and it will inflame your skin as you brush.

▲ 1 feet and lower legs

- Take the brush and begin with the sole of your left foot. Use firm rhythmic strokes to cover the sole several times.

- Next, brush the top of your foot, brushing upwards towards your ankle.

- Move on to your lower leg, brushing the entire surface in a series of upwards strokes.

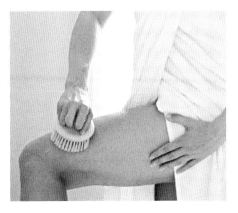

▲ 2 upper legs

• Stand up straight and brush the area from your knee to the top of your thigh. Brush your buttock area as far up as your waist.

• Repeat the procedure on the other leg.

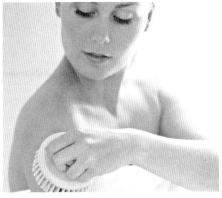

▲ 3 back and shoulders

• Moving in an upward direction, brush your back several times from your buttocks all the way up to your shoulders.

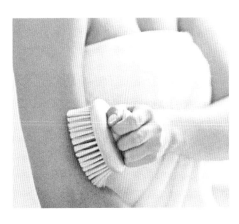

▲ 4 arms

• Next brush your right arm. Start with the palm of your hand, move up the back and then brush from your wrist up to your elbow, again in an upward direction.

• Brush your upper arm from your elbow up to the shoulder, covering the whole surface several times in a series of strokes.

• Repeat the procedure on the left arm.

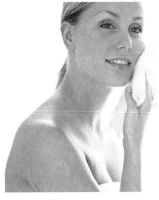

▲ 5 neck and chest

• The neck and chest are sensitive areas so brush lightly here, again always moving in the direction of the heart.

• Once you have finished brushing, shower or at least rinse the skin.

massage

When many of us think of massage for cellulite, we think of intense, pummelling massage. Recent research suggests this probably isn't a good idea. While a professional massage therapist may be able to use the right amount of force to massage in this way, most of us pinch and pummel too forcefully or use the wrong motions. This actually damages the septa, which need to be repaired. Harsh movements can also damage the flow of lymph, causing further stagnation.

The right type of massage, however, can be incredibly powerful. According to Chinese researchers, when the body is massaged, the temperature of the skin increases. This widens the gaps between the cells of the body, allowing lymph to flow more easily.

So what is the right type of massage for cellulite? The most beneficial is called manual lymph drainage and uses a mixture of long gentle strokes with pulsing techniques to focus on stimulating the flow of lymph.

Full manual lymph drainage must always be carried out by a specialist or the lymphatic system can be damaged, so ask at your nearest health store or health centre for recommendations. However, you can carry out a very gentle form of lymph massage yourself.

Make sure that you keep your strokes long and gentle, so that you don't cause any damage to your septa or lymph.

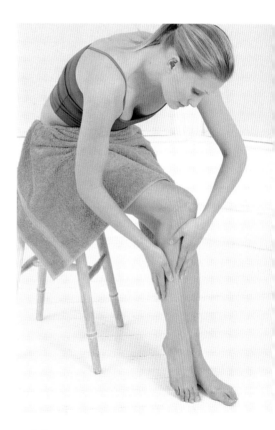

▲ 1 legs

- Start on your legs, with long gentle strokes from the ankles, moving upwards towards the knees. Work both the front and back of the leg.

- Then move up the thighs, with long strokes front and back towards the groin.

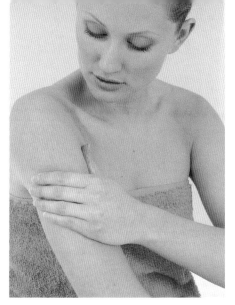

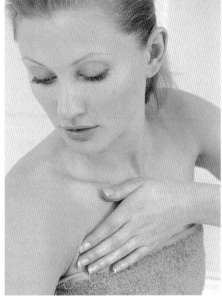

▲ 2 arms

- Work around the arms upwards from wrists to elbows.
- Now move past the elbows, massaging the upper arms towards the armpits.

▲ 3 upper body

- Next massage your upper torso with the same long strokes.
- Massage outwards and either upwards or downwards towards your armpits, depending on which area you are massaging.
- If someone is massaging your back, they should direct the strokes on the upper back and shoulder blades towards your armpits; the neck strokes should go towards the ears.

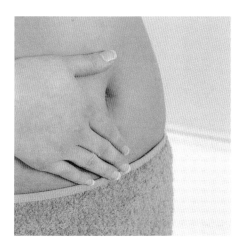

◀ 4 lower abdomen

- Lastly work the lower abdomen. The area under your navel should be massaged towards the groin.
- If someone is massaging your back, then the strokes should go upwards and around the hips.

heat and water treatments

Heat and water treatments include saunas, steams and hydrotherapy, which can dramatically boost circulation. In fact, during a sauna, blood flow from the heart increases by up to 75 per cent, and 70 per cent of that blood reaches the skin. Any toxins carried in the blood are therefore closer to the surface of the body and, so the theory goes, will be more likely to be excreted in the sweat, relieving some of the pressure from your lymph system.

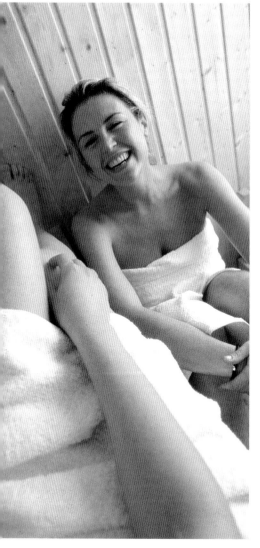

STEAMS AND SAUNAS

While devotees claim that saunas of 2–3 hours can break down fat stores and help eliminate cellulite entirely, it should not be done without medical supervision. You will get just as positive a result by spending 10–20 minutes at a time at a temperature you can bear. Don't eat a heavy meal or drink alcohol before the treatment, but do drink plenty of water before, during and after your session. You can lose 25 g (1 oz) of water or more in a sauna, which is enough to make you dehydrated.

If you are pregnant or have any medical problems that involve your heart, blood pressure, respiratory system or skin, see your doctor before having saunas or steams to check if they are safe.

HYDROTHERAPY

Hydrotherapy is the therapeutic use of water, and can include baths, showers and water-based massage treatments. Like massage and skin brushing, most hydrotherapy treatments aim to boost the circulation and lymph flow, by using either the force of the water or changes in temperature. However, new research shows that hydrotherapy may even encourage weight loss. According to a study published in the *New England Journal of Medicine*, diabetic patients who soaked in a hot tub for 30 minutes a day, six days a week for three weeks, actually lost an average of 1.7 kg (3¾ lb) each.

There are many ways you can harness the power of hydrotherapy, the easiest of which is a hydrotherapy bath, which uses the pressure of water from a showerhead for massage. For this you will need a bath with a shower hose that can reach under the water. If your showerhead is attached to the wall, buy a shower hose that will hook temporarily on to a tap.

Remember always to work towards the heart as you move the showerhead up your legs. If you have heart problems, reduce the temperature of the water very gradually from warm to cold. If you are prone to broken veins, keep the water pressure low and the water just on warm.

If you don't have a bath, it doesn't mean you can't use hydrotherapy. Just finish each shower with a 2–3-minute warm water massage with the showerhead on the highest pressure you can bear, then follow up with a 1–2-minute blast of cold.

WHAT TO DO WHEN

treatment	when to do it
skin brushing	every day before a bath or shower
manual lymph massage	once a week
steams/saunas	once a week
hydrotherapy bath	at least three times a week

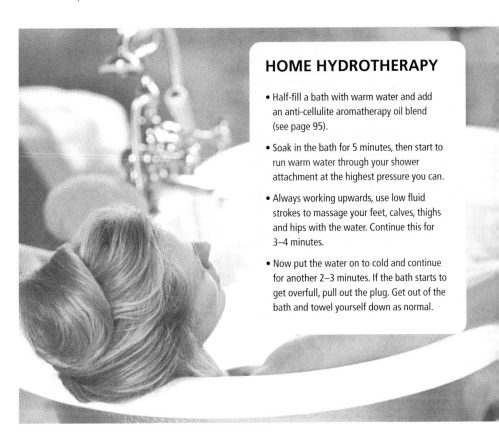

HOME HYDROTHERAPY

- Half-fill a bath with warm water and add an anti-cellulite aromatherapy oil blend (see page 95).

- Soak in the bath for 5 minutes, then start to run warm water through your shower attachment at the highest pressure you can.

- Always working upwards, use low fluid strokes to massage your feet, calves, thighs and hips with the water. Continue this for 3–4 minutes.

- Now put the water on to cold and continue for another 2–3 minutes. If the bath starts to get overfull, pull out the plug. Get out of the bath and towel yourself down as normal.

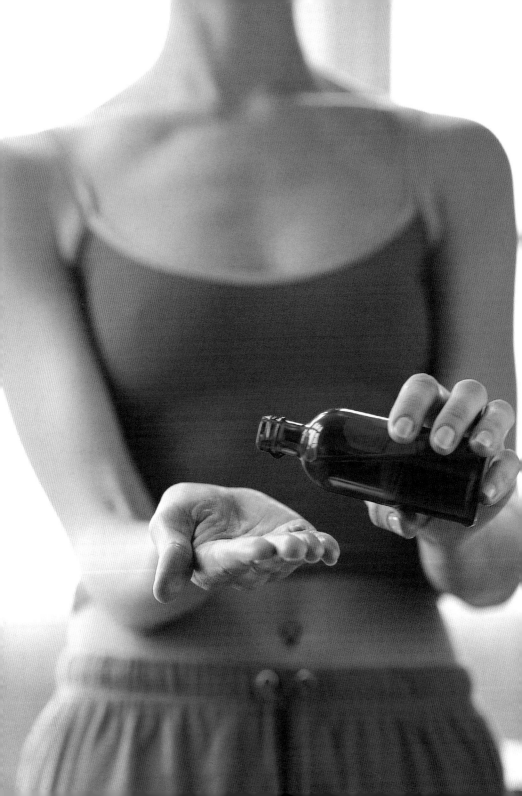

the aromatherapy solution

The Aromatherapy Solution uses the natural power of essential oils to fight cellulite. These are concentrated oils made directly from the roots, flowers, fruits, seeds, stalks or leaves of a plant. The oil of a plant includes many of the same elements and has the same effects as the whole plant – orange oil, for example, contains vitamin C just like the fruit, while spicy black-pepper oil creates the same warming feeling on the body as peppercorns do on the tongue. These properties mean that aromatherapy oils can have potent physical or mental benefits.

The Aromatherapy Solution focuses on oils that play a part in reducing cellulite, and they work in a number of different ways. Many oils are diuretic, helping to reduce the amount of excess fluid stored; some boost circulation and help to stimulate blood flow and the lymph; other oils have skin-strengthening properties and maximize the healthy regeneration of collagen. There are also other elements that may help more indirectly by lowering the appetite or fighting stress which may trigger comfort-eating or increase fat storage. Combining a mixture of these properties in oil blends can therefore help speed the elimination of cellulite through a variety of means.

The other benefit of aromatherapy is that it is one of the most pleasurable solutions to cellulite. What could be nicer than sinking into a bath full of wonderfully scented warm water, or more indulgent than having someone soothe your body with a massage?

CONTENTS

using aromatherapy

Essential oils can be used in a whole host of ways, from oil burners that scent rooms to direct application on to the skin. When it comes to fighting cellulite, however, massage, bathing and inhalation are the most effective ways of using oils.

MASSAGE

By applying essential oils directly to the skin through massage you can concentrate the power of the oil in the area you most want to treat – in this case the hips, thighs and buttocks. However, essential oils should not be used neat on the skin as they can cause irritation or even be toxic. Instead, mix them with a 'carrier' oil first, which will carry the essential oil safely on to the skin.

There are a whole host of carrier oils on the market, but grapeseed oil is particularly suited to fighting cellulite as it contains high levels of

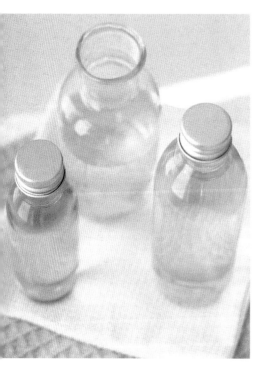

antioxidants, which strengthen the skin. However, whichever oil you use, the rule is the same: use half the number of drops of essential oil as there are millilitres of carrier oil in the bottle. For example, add a total of 12 or 13 drops of essential oils to a 25 ml (1 fl oz) bottle of carrier oil.

After you have mixed the oil, use a small palmful to massage each leg, using long sweeping motions up towards the groin. See page 88 for a fuller massage.

BATHING

This is the simplest way to use aromatherapy, as the oils are absorbed into the skin while you soak. You will get maximum benefit if you run your bath, then sprinkle 3–6 drops of essential oil on the surface. Agitate the water to ensure you don't get a concentrated dose on your skin. You can use aromatherapy blends as part of a hydrotherapy bath (see page 91).

INHALATIONS

These are normally used to treat stress or headaches, but they can have a small part to play in fighting cellulite by helping with motivation or cravings and stress control. The easiest way to use inhalations is to place 3–4 drops of oil on a tissue and breathe in deeply for 5–10 breaths.

BLENDING OILS

Mix and match some of the oils overleaf with the properties you'd like to harness most, or try some of the following blends.

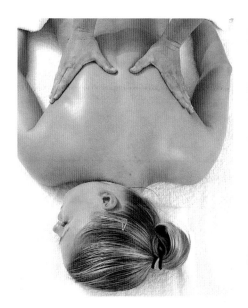

WHAT TO DO WHEN

How often you should use the oils depends upon which method you choose to apply them – massage contains a more concentrated dose than bathing.

treatment	when to do it
massage	1–3 times a week
bath	daily
inhalations	when you need them, no more than 2–3 times a day

Fluid fighter

Use on soft, spongy cellulite or if fluid is likely to be a major cause of your cellulite.
- 1 drop of fennel
- 1 drop of cypress
- 1 drop of grapefruit
- 2 drops of juniper

Add to 10ml of carrier oil and use for massage or bathing.

Skin firmer

Use on mature skin, or as a preventative once you have lost weight/fluid from your cellulite.
- 2 drops of neroli
- 2 drops of carrot seed
- 1 drop of orange

Mix with 10ml of carrier oil and use for massage.

Diet aider

Use to aid fat burning and help reduce food cravings.
- 1 drop of black pepper
- 1 drop of patchouli
- 2 drops of geranium
- 1 drop of neroli

Mix with 10ml of carrier oil and use for massage or bathing. Inhale to suppress hunger.

AROMATHERAPY TIPS

• Essential oils can be very potent, so do not exceed the recommended dose.

• Patch-test all oils before you use them by applying a tiny amount to the skin on the inside of your arm. If you get any stinging, irritation or reddening, then don't use that oil.

• Some oils can interfere with medical conditions including epilepsy and diabetes. If you have a medical condition, seek advice from a registered aromatherapist before treating yourself.

• Many oils are not suitable for pregnant women. Ask for professional advice.

• Essential oils should never be taken internally.

top 10 anti-cellulite oils

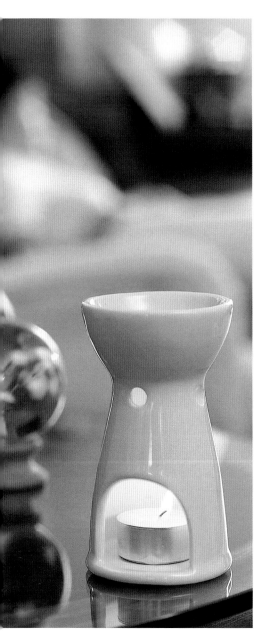

1 CYPRESS

A potent fluid-reducer, this pine-scented oil is important if your cellulite has a spongy, waterlogged feel or look. It also helps regulate circulation and is very good for other problems associated with circulation, such as varicose veins. It seems to have hormone-balancing properties, which may counteract some of the oestrogen-related elements of cellulite.
Take care: Avoid during pregnancy.
Blends well with: juniper, lemon, orange

2 GERANIUM

Strongly floral, this oil detoxifies the body from within. It is a good diuretic and helps stimulate both liver and kidneys. It boosts the immune system, stimulates the lymphatic system and thins the blood, making circulation more efficient. Geranium also balances the body mentally – calming you when you are stressed and energizing you when you are feeling tired.
Take care: Avoid during pregnancy. Always test on your skin first.
Blends well with: carrot seed, grapefruit, neroli, orange

3 NEROLI

A very important skin oil, it helps regenerate damaged skin cells and improves elasticity and hydration of the skin. Neroli is often used to treat stretch marks, which frequently come hand in hand with cellulite. A circulation booster, neroli also helps tackle problems like broken capillaries. Finally, the ethereal, floral scent of neroli is good for helping relieve stress – and the resulting muscle tension and potential weight gain that can be related to this.
Blends well with: geranium, lemon, orange

4 ORANGE

Orange oil helps the body absorb vitamin C, which is vital to fight free-radical damage and can reinforce the natural processes that lead to collagen formation. It boosts bile flow within the liver and therefore may help with fat digestion, but like most citrus oils it also stimulates the appetite. If the skin is congested, it will encourage it to sweat, which helps reduce toxins held under the surface and may aid the lymph.

Blends well with: cypress, geranium, juniper

5 GRAPEFRUIT

This is a fat-fighting oil as it helps stimulate bile production in the liver, and it is bile that helps your body process fat. It also stimulates the lymph system and helps balance fluid levels. It has an energizing and uplifting effect on the mind, which makes it good if you are getting fed up with following diet or exercise plans. However, it can increase the appetite.

Take care: Don't expose your skin to the sun after using grapefruit oil.

Blends well with: geranium

6 CARROT SEED

This oil is an excellent skin toner, which can be used as part of body-firming massage treatments. It helps reduce fluid retention and boost red blood cells, increasing the amount of oxygen reaching body tissues and the fibroblasts within them. It also helps fight feelings of stress and exhaustion. Try a sniff (it has quite a sweet scent) if you need to calm down and de-stress, or if you want to energize yourself before your workout.

Take care: Avoid during pregnancy.

Blends well with: juniper, lemon, neroli, orange

7 FENNEL

If you are having trouble sticking to your diet, fennel suppresses the appetite (although liquorice lovers may find its aniseed scent a temptation). It also helps fight fluid retention and detoxifies the body. Fennel may have antioxidant properties as it is used as a cure for

wrinkles and cataracts, both of which are linked to exposure to free radicals.

Take care: Avoid during pregnancy, or if you have epilepsy. Always test on your skin first.

Blends well with: geranium, lemon

8 JUNIPER

Juniper helps detoxify the body, taking pressure off the lymph system, and also helps fight fluid retention. It is an appetite regulator, so inhale a few drops on a tissue to help reduce food cravings.

Take care: Stick to the stated dose: too much juniper can stimulate the kidneys to work too hard, overtaxing them. Avoid during pregnancy.

Blends well with: cypress, geranium, grapefruit, orange

9 BLACK PEPPER

With its spicy warming scent, black pepper is a good circulation enhancer, dilating blood vessels in the area in which it is applied. It also has a diuretic effect and is believed to help the body digest proteins, a major part of the anti-cellulite diet. It can also help tone muscles.

Take care: Never use it neat on the skin and only ever use 1–2 drops in massage or bath blends, as it can irritate.

Blends well with: cypress, geranium, grapefruit, lemon

10 PATCHOULI

This is the oil for dieters. It curbs appetite, but also clarifies the mind if you are not sure about something (like whether to have that slice of chocolate cake). A diuretic oil, it helps fight fluid retention, but also helps tone and firm the skin. Finally, patchouli acts directly on the skin cells, stimulating growth and healing of the connective fibres. Its exotic fragrance makes it very much an evening oil, but some people cannot stand the scent.

Blends well with: black pepper, geranium, neroli

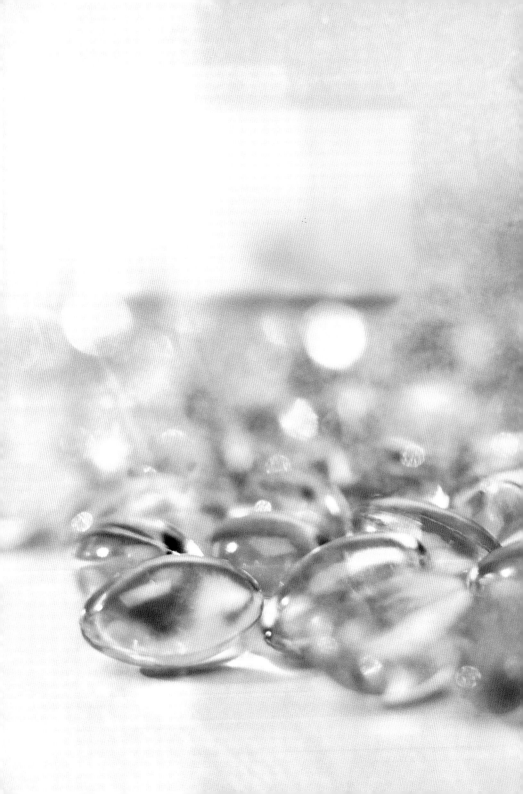

the supplement solution

While the Diet Solution can work wonders at removing cellulite on its own, you can increase its effects even further by using herbal or nutrient supplements, or even natural herbs that you may already be using in your cooking. These can have fat-fighting, fluid-busting and skin-strengthening properties, and it's these that we are going to explore in the Supplement Solution.

It would be nice to think these supplements would work on their own and that you won't have to follow the diet and exercise programmes. However, whatever some supplement manufacturers claim, there is not a magic pill that will cure cellulite. Pills have been launched that claim to remove cellulite, but independent trials do not show the same success rates the manufacturers claim. In fact, when researchers at South Bank University, London, tested one pill, the subjects actually gained weight, possibly because they thought that with their cellulite being controlled by miracle means, it didn't matter what they ate or how much they exercised.

Instead of a complete cure, the role of the Supplement Solution is to supplement all the benefits you are achieving from the other Solutions. Over the next few pages, you will find seven really important pills or potions that you should consider taking in relatively large quantities, plus a whole host of herbs that can be integrated in small daily doses (should you so desire) into the foods you are eating. This doesn't mean you should take them all, however. Something you don't need could cause reactions in the body that hinder rather than help your cellulite. For example, should you take diuretic dandelion when you don't have excess fluid, you may cause dehydration, which could panic your body into retaining more fluids. Instead, there are two supplements that should be taken by everyone throughout the programme, and the others should only be used if you think you need their benefits.

CONTENTS

the seven superfighters

These are the most important supplements and herbs you should be taking to help fight cellulite. While many of them can be found naturally in your diet, by taking them in supplement form, you can take in more concentrated doses that will ensure you are really getting the benefits. But remember, don't take them all, just those most relevant to you.

1 ANTIOXIDANTS

Maximizing your intake of antioxidants is an important part of the anti-cellulite programme. The main way to do this is with food: researchers are pretty sure that antioxidants need other, undetermined ingredients in fruits and vegetables to work to their full advantage. However, if your diet is good, supplementing will only enhance the effects. The best anti-cellulite nutrients (and those safe in high levels) are vitamin C and vitamin E.

WHAT TO TAKE:
Take 3 g of vitamin C (the most your body can store) in three equal doses each day. Take 400iu of vitamin E each day.

2 GOTU KOLA

Scientifically known as *Centella asiatica*, this herb is traditionally used to help wounds heal faster. In clinical trials it has been shown to increase the formation of new collagen, good news for cellulite sufferers wanting to keep their septa strong. Italian researchers have also found that doses of the herb can improve circulation and reduce fluid retention in people suffering from weak veins.

WHAT TO TAKE:
Take 30 mg three times each day.

3 CONJUGATED LINOLEIC ACID (CLA)

Commonly found in meat and dairy products, this fatty acid has now been shown by four independent studies to increase the amount of body fat burnt during diet and exercise – and to increase the amount of lean muscle mass (which will help disguise cellulite) in the system. In one trial carried out by Swedish researchers at the University of Uppsala, patients taking CLA

for 14 weeks lost 3.8 per cent of their body fat.

WHAT TO TAKE:
If you need to lose body fat, take two 500 mg capsules of CLA three times each day with meals.

4 GINKGO BILOBA

This was one of the major components of the cellulite miracle pill, and is also an extremely common ingredient in many anti-cellulite creams. The reason is that it increases the rate of blood flow around the body, by up to 57 per cent according to one German study. Ginkgo also has antioxidant properties. It is good if you have poor circulation, if you are often cold when others are warm or can feel particularly cold patches within your areas of cellulite.

WHAT TO TAKE:
If you need to improve your circulation, take 170 mg a day throughout the programme. If you get headaches, reduce your dose by half until symptoms stop.

5 GREEN TEA

As well as being an antioxidant, green tea has been shown to increase the rate at which we burn calories. Drinking three cups a day will help you burn an extra 80 calories in the next 24 hours. That adds up to a weight loss of 2.8 kg (6 lb) a year. Green tea may also reduce weight by stopping the production of fat-absorbing enzymes. According to French researchers, you could lose 30 per cent of your fat calories a day simply by drinking more.

WHAT TO TAKE:
If you are trying to lose weight, add two green tea pills or at least three cups of green tea to your daily diet (remember herbal teas can replace glasses of water in your daily allowance).

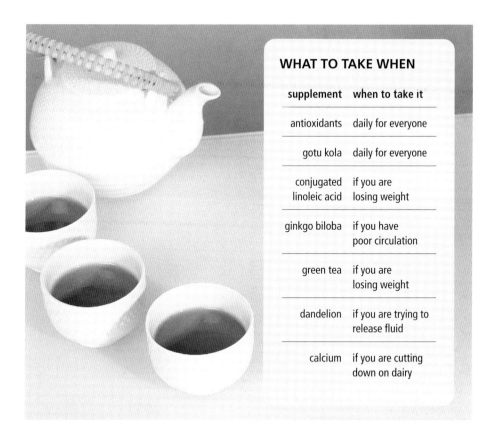

WHAT TO TAKE WHEN

supplement	when to take it
antioxidants	daily for everyone
gotu kola	daily for everyone
conjugated linoleic acid	if you are losing weight
ginkgo biloba	if you have poor circulation
green tea	if you are losing weight
dandelion	if you are trying to release fluid
calcium	if you are cutting down on dairy

6 DANDELION

If fluid plays a part in your cellulite, this diuretic herb will help release trapped fluid in the system – but safely. Many diuretics cause the body to leach vital potassium stores from the body with excess water, which upsets fluid balance further – and, more seriously, is bad for your heart. Dandelion is the exception to this as it actually contains high levels of potassium and therefore helps fight fluid without causing harm elsewhere. Dandelion is also high in antioxidants.

WHAT TO TAKE:

Dandelion supplements can be found in health stores and are thought by most people to be the most palatable way to use the herb. If you like bitter tastes, you can also add fresh dandelion leaves to an ordinary salad or drink the tea. Aim for three cups each day.

7 CALCIUM

If you are cutting out dairy products as part of your diet, it is vital that you supplement with calcium during the programme. High levels of calcium are essential for women in their twenties and thirties to help them build bone, and vital for women older than this to help prevent bone loss. On top of this, studies at the University of Tennessee have shown calcium to be a vital fat-fighting nutrient – in trials it was found that increasing calcium levels in the diet increases fat loss by 60 per cent.

WHAT TO TAKE:

If you are cutting down on dairy, supplement with 1,000 mg of calcium each day.

spice up your life

Herbs and spices are something most of us use every day to flavour food, but they also have potent health-giving properties. So, by choosing cellulite-fighting herbs or spices when you cook, you can boost the effects of the cellulite-busting foods that you eat. Look through the list and find the ones that will best tackle your cellulite.

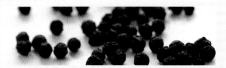

BLACK PEPPER
An antioxidant, black pepper also helps prevent the depletion of the vital detoxifying enzyme glutathione in the body, which is good news for your lymph. Black pepper boosts circulation and is believed to stimulate the metabolism – although it also stimulates the appetite, so watch how much you use in any one go.
Foods it goes well with: almost anything

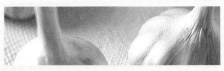

GARLIC
High in sulphur compounds, garlic helps boost detoxification in the body. Garlic also helps keep blood vessels supple, boosting circulation. It contains vital ingredients called ajoenes that thin the blood, again improving your circulation. Garlic is also a source of the vital antioxidant selenium that powers up the skin-boosting antioxidant vitamins A,C and E.
Foods it goes well with: almost anything

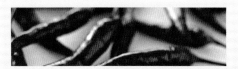

CHILLI
A potent metabolism booster (something shown by the perspiration that occurs when you eat it), chilli has been shown to increase the speed at which we burn calories by up to 10 per cent. As well as this, chilli may also suppress the appetite. Scientists at Quebec's Laval University found that after adding spicy condiments (like Tabasco or chilli sauce) to one meal, women ate considerably less at the next.
Foods it goes well with: fish, chicken, eggs, tofu

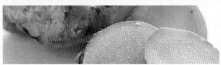

GINGER
Known for boosting peripheral circulation, ginger is another metabolism-boosting herb (something signified by its slightly spicy taste). On top of this, it is an antioxidant, containing 21 different ingredients that fight free radicals.
Foods it goes well with: fish, chicken, sushi

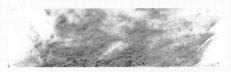

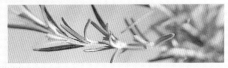

TURMERIC

Used in Ayurvedic medicine to help reduce fluid, turmeric is also an antioxidant. On top of this, its spicy taste makes it a metabolic booster and potentially an appetite suppressant. Ayurvedic wisdom also claims that turmeric boosts energy levels, good for anyone on the Exercise Solution.
Foods it goes well with: chicken, beef, fish, eggs

ROSEMARY

Rosemary is well known for fighting the capillary fragility that can cause fluid to leak into the surrounding tissues, and is an extremely important anti-cellulite herb. It is therefore included in many brands of anti-cellulite cream. It is also an antioxidant and detoxifying herb.
Foods it goes well with: lamb, beef, chicken, fish

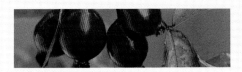

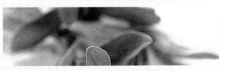

ROSEHIPS

Although rosehips are known for their high levels of vitamin C, they are also rich in the B vitamins, other antioxidants and carotenoids. Rosewater and rose oil are vital skin-strengthening ingredients and it is thought that rosehips can also boost healthy skin.
Foods it goes well with: most commonly used as a tea, but rosehip syrup or jelly can also be used on toast or crackers (it does contain sugar, so use sparingly)

MARJORAM

Used as an energizing herb, marjoram is another diuretic. It also helps regulate the bowel, which is good news, as a sluggish bowel can lead to toxins waiting to be expelled being reabsorbed, increasing the risk of allergies, food intolerances and an overworked lymph system.
Foods it goes well with: meat, oily fish, tomatoes, peppers, aubergines

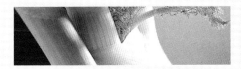

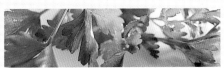

FENNEL

This is a very diuretic herb and the seeds sprinkled on a salad can help boost the fluid-balancing power of vegetables like celery or cucumber. Fennel is also used as an appetite suppresser and so could be helpful if you are finding your diet difficult.
Foods it goes well with: fish, lamb

PARSLEY

A good kidney tonic, parsley can help beat fluid retention. It is also a powerful antioxidant and rich in vitamin C. Adding one cup of leaves to a salad, for example, would provide your entire recommended daily intake of vitamin C.
Foods it goes well with: fish, salads, cottage cheese, jacket potatoes

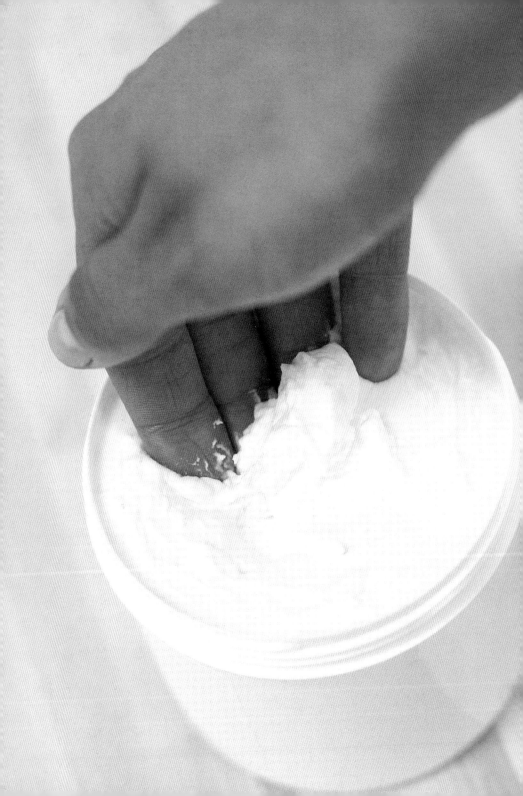

the
beauty solution

If there is one thing most of us want when it comes to cellulite, it is a quick fix. We want it gone and we want it gone now, and that's where the Beauty Solution helps. While it is the Diet and Exercise Solutions that offer the biggest benefit in fighting the fat, and the other Solutions help cement those benefits in the long term, you will have to wait at least two or three weeks before you see any results, and at least six before you end up with a finished product. The Beauty Solution's primary job, however, is to make you feel better about the way your hips and thighs look now. This is the one Solution that will reduce the look of your cellulite within 24 hours.

Just as there is no miracle pill, there's no miracle cream, however. What you are primarily doing is disguising the look of the cellulite until the other Solutions can get to work. But while this quick-fix element of the Beauty Solution is a distinct benefit, it doesn't mean the whole Solution is just a smokescreen. No one group of people is working harder to find a cure for cellulite than the beauty industry and never before have there been so many ingredients that are being shown

to fight it. On every high street you can now find creams that truly can help reduce fluid, that are proven to increase the elasticity and health of the skin, and that may even encourage the burning of fat. The Beauty Solution explains how to find these products and how to use them to maximum advantage. And finally, we will be looking at the most hi-tech element of cellulite fighting, the salon treatments, and discovering exactly what they deliver, to help you decide if you want to make them part of your cellulite-fighting plan.

CONTENTS

moisturizing and cellulite creams

It's a simple beauty truth that most women think their skincare regime should stop at their neck, and their bodies get a lick of body lotion only once in a while. However, the skin on our bodies is even more likely than our faces to get dehydrated, and this can make cellulite appear much worse than it actually is.

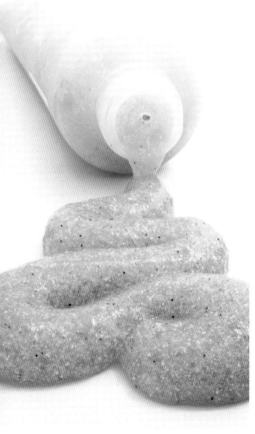

While most of us would be horrified at the idea of using soap and water on our faces, we happily step into baths full of bubbles. Bubblebath is just as likely to dry out the skin, and we tend to soak for too long in too-hot water. As a result, our body skin is usually chronically dehydrated. In terms of cellulite, this is bad news. Dehydrated skin is more prone to cellulite, as UV rays penetrate deeper and trigger more collagen and elastin damage. Dehydrated skin looks duller, which means light is absorbed into it and highlights any defects. Also, dry skin is thinner than it should be, just enough for the fat cells underneath to be more noticeable.

The rapid results of the Beauty Solution are primarily down to rehydration. By simply moisturizing your skin morning and night, you will plump up the upper layer and create a slightly thicker layer between your cellulite and the outside world. However, it is possible to enhance the hydration effect by using products with particular ingredients.

CELLULITE CREAMS

Replacing your body lotion once a day with a cream that has some kind of anti-cellulite ingredients will mean you are not just getting the benefit of rehydration, but are also tackling the causes of cellulite. Cellulite creams contain a myriad of ingredients, some of which are more effective than others. The following three ingredients seem to be the most beneficial.

aminophylline

This was first developed to reduce the symptoms of asthma, but two doctors reported that when women had treated one thigh with the cream, that thigh shrank. They argued that aminophylline entered the cells and caused the fat to break down. Other trials have disputed the results, but companies still working with aminophylline claim the reason other trials have

FAKE TAN

Tanning your skin is another way to quickly reduce the dimple effect by simply making the bumps less noticeable and making you feel better about your appearance. However, as we saw on page 15, sunbathing is the most detrimental thing you can do to your skin, so fake tan is the answer. If you choose a good-quality product and take time to apply it properly, you can disguise your cellulite in a matter of hours.

not worked is that, once the fat is released into the bloodstream, it won't disappear on its own – you have to exercise to burn it off. On the exercise programme this won't be an issue. If you buy a cream containing aminophylline, keep it away from heat and use it quickly.

centella asiatica

You may recognize this from the supplement section, and just as studies have shown that this herb (also known as gotu kola) may help cellulite from inside, topical application also seems to give results. Research trials have proven that it increases new collagen in an area. It is also claimed to help strengthen the fibroblasts, preventing them from acting abnormally in cellulite tissue. Last but not least, it can have diuretic properties.

retinol

A derivative of the antioxidant vitamin A, retinol is commonly used in anti-wrinkle creams. It works by speeding cell renewal (which makes the skin behave more youthfully) and by increasing the rate of collagen production. It has been shown to improve the elasticity of the skin by about 10 per cent after six months of treatment. This frees up the septa and loosens the skin over the protruding fat cells, reducing the doming effect of the cellulite.

ADDED EXTRAS

These ingredients will also boost the effects of any cream.

Butcher's broom (*Ruscus aculeatus*) This herb has been shown to improve circulation to the lower limbs. It also has a mild diuretic action.

Caffeine Caffeine is one of the main ingredients in anti-cellulite creams. Like aminophylline, caffeine helps release fat from the fat stores. However, bear in mind that caffeine is diuretic and will tone and firm the skin by reducing the water within it, as well as fighting fat.

Horse chestnut (*Aesculus hippocastanum*) This helps boost blood flow, strengthens the veins and capillaries and can help prevent or lessen the effects of varicose veins. It is also a fluid fighter.

Ivy (*Hedera helix*) This reduces fluid retention and will make your thighs marginally firmer and thinner. However, ivy can have quite a high allergy risk. If you have sensitive skin, patch-test on a small area for a few days before using it all over your legs.

Menthol This cooling gel is said to increase circulation. As well as this, the coolness constricts the skin, firming and toning the thighs.

USING CREAMS

If you want to get the best results from your cellulite cream you need to time things right. If you have a once-a-day cream, it is usually best to apply it at night, as skin is more permeable at night and any active ingredients are more likely to be drawn in. The night-time approach is even more important if your cream contains retinol, as this is destroyed by exposure to light. To prevent the cream being washed off, use it after your bath or shower on dry skin, so the ingredients have the maximum amount of time to absorb. Apply it using light, upward strokes – rather like a mini lymph drainage (see page 88).

salon treatments

As well as the numerous beauty products, there is a whole host of salon treatments that claim to treat cellulite. With one noticeable exception, their main role is to make the cellulite less noticeable by plumping up or firming the skin on a short-term basis. Whether you use salon treatments or not is up to you: they aren't essential to get results and, in many cases, the cost of having enough treatments to see a difference will be huge. However, here are the most popular – or most promising – salon-based cellulite treatments.

CELLULITE MASSAGES

These combine diuretic products or oils with massage techniques, usually those used in manual lymphatic drainage (see page 88). In the right hands, at the end of a one-hour treatment you will end up with smoother skin and a loss of fluid from the fatty tissue. Continued usage should help reduce the stagnation of the lymph and therefore stop cellulite getting worse. For best results, however, you should visit someone specifically trained in manual lymph drainage.

GEL WRAPS

Therapeutic gels are smeared over the body and you are wrapped in heat-inducing blankets so that you can sweat. The gel ingredients vary, though seaweed and mud are common. These are packed with minerals, which means they have a negative electrical charge. The skin is positively charged, so the minerals are drawn into the skin, which causes a balancing of the fluid levels in your body. Dry areas are hydrated and waterlogged areas (like your cellulite) give up some of their excess fluid.

Menthol-based gels turn the area cold and aim to temporarily tighten the skin and boost circulation within the hips and thighs. At the end of the treatment your skin will look and feel smoother and firmer. Both types of wrap do help reduce fluid levels, so if fluid is a big part of your problem they will help, but to really make an impact you need weekly treatments.

Take care: If you are allergic to shellfish, do not have seaweed wraps as they can trigger an allergic reaction. They should also be avoided by anyone with a thyroid condition.

BANDAGE WRAPS

Like gel wraps, these use seaweed or menthol gels, but rather than wrapping you in a warm blanket, your therapist wraps you tightly in cloth or plastic bandages. This helps constrict the tissues and may encourage more fluid to be lost. However, fluid loss is all that's happening. Some advertisments claim to help you lose 7 cm (3 inches) in one session, but that is frequently calculated by taking measurements in 15 different places and adding up all the tiny losses. However, if fluid is a major part of your cellulite problem, regular treatments can make a noticeable difference.

ELECTRICAL TREATMENTS

This takes the seaweed cure one step further. Rather than just applying the gel and letting it work its way into the skin, electrical treatments use tiny electrodes placed on the skin to charge it. The idea is that this extra charge forces the products deeper into the skin than they would normally go. Some treatments also use another type of charge, which 'exercises' the thigh muscles while the cream does its work, firming and lifting the thighs and buttocks. Again, it will make a difference after one treatment – and a course may slightly lift the muscles, firming the buttocks.

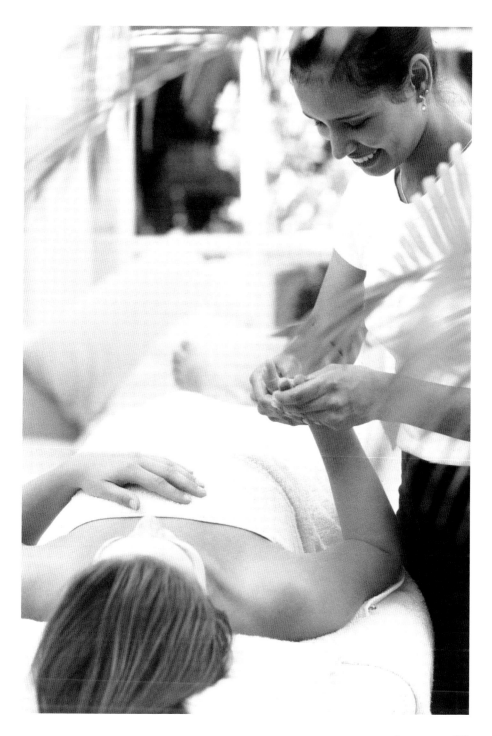

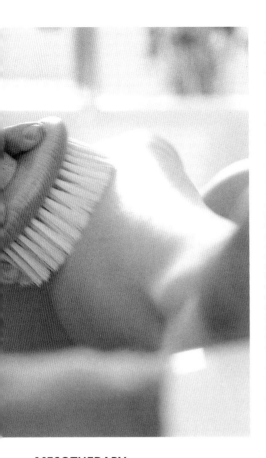

CAN COSMETIC SURGERY ACTUALLY HELP?

At the moment the answer to this question is no. Liposuction is a treatment where the fatty tissue under the skin is broken up and then sucked out of the body. While exceptionally good at removing inches and slimming down hips, thighs and buttocks, it doesn't deal with the damaged septa in the area, so it doesn't actually get rid of cellulite. And while the removal of the fat cells guarantees you won't put on weight in that area again, if you don't watch your weight the fat will have to go somewhere – creating cellulite on your tummy perhaps?

However, cosmetic surgery techniques are being refined every day and liposuction techniques are being combined with keyhole surgery procedures that cut the septa in the area where the liposuction is being carried out. Good results are also being shown from liposuction patients who have endermologie treatments after liposuction. However, bear in mind that any surgical procedure has risks and should never be undertaken lightly. Liposuction should really be a last resort as a way to treat cellulite – or any kind of weight gain.

MESOTHERAPY

In this treatment, an analysis is made to determine what might be causing the cellulite and doses of remedies for that cause are injected just under the skin, very quickly, rather like a tattoo needle. For example, if poor circulation is to blame, a circulation-boosting treatment would be used; if lymph is the main problem, a lymph-boosting and strengthening product would be used. Vitamin C is also sometimes included to boost collagen production. Many patients receive a cocktail of treatments, generally using natural products – gotu kola, for example, is a common addition to treatments. Once- or twice-weekly treatments over 4–8 weeks are recommended. You then have a 4-week maintenance course once a year. Practitioners claim to be able to reduce cellulite by 40–50 per cent over 3–4

treatments, and perhaps eventually get rid of it altogether. It must be carried out by someone with medical training and in most countries (except France) availability is limited.

ENDERMOLOGIE

This technique has been used in France since the 1980s, but only really made big news when the US Food and Drug Administration approved it as a treatment that temporarily reduces the look and feel of cellulite. The treatment uses a

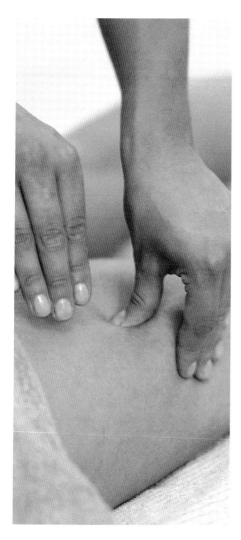

their thighs after seven treatments. However, it is not cheap and the minimum number of treatments required is ten, with twice-yearly maintenance sessions to keep up results.

ULTRASOUND MASSAGES

This relatively new treatment uses ultrasound waves to reputedly blast the fat cells and dissolve them. The newly released fat is then passed into the bloodstream and harmlessly excreted out of the system. This method appeared as a side effect of a new liposuction technique that uses sound waves to break down the fat instead of the normal manual method (the idea being that it reduces the bruising). Of course in liposuction the fat is actually sucked out of the system and removed – the concern about ultrasound is where the fat ends up. Is it reabsorbed, passed out or does it attach itself to the insides of the arteries? Further trials will be carried out on this treatment over the next few years.

WHAT TO DO WHEN

treatment	when to do it
body lotion	after a bath or shower (if you are doing an aromatherapy treatment, skip your lotion)
fake tan	the first or second day you start the programme and every 3–4 days after that
anti-cellulite creams	every night
salon treatments	once a week or as recommended by your practitioner (if you want to)

mixture of suction and rollers to massage the fat cells intensely, breaking them down. It also boosts circulation, which, it is claimed, causes the broken-down fat to be carried out of the system. However, what makes endermologie truly different is that the rollers also stretch the septa, preventing them from pulling down on the skin and creating the doming that occurs with cellulite. It has been shown to work – one trial published in the *Aesthetic Surgery Journal* found women lost 1.34 cm (about ½ inch) from

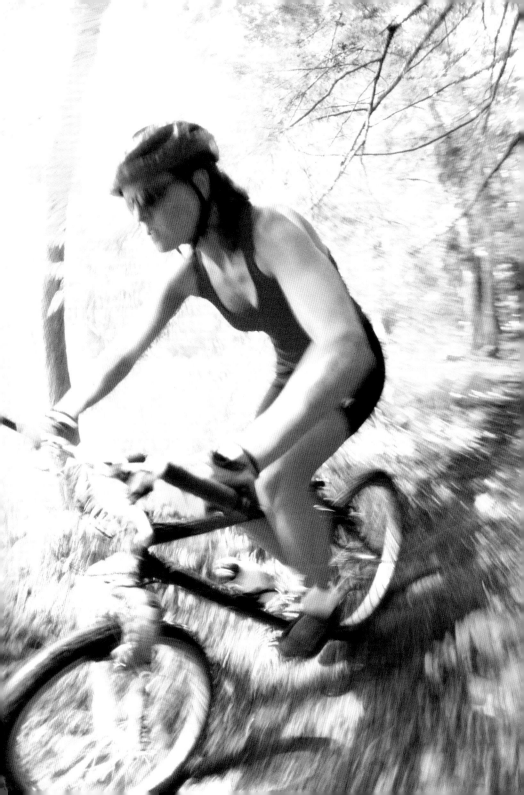

the
psychological
solution

So far we have concentrated on the physical elements of cellulite; the point of the Psychological Solution is to give yourself a big mental makeover. Even though cellulite is a purely physical problem, a positive mental attitude will maximize the chances of the whole process succeeding. According to research by the US National Weight Control Registry, 82 per cent of those who had successfully managed to lose weight after failing before said the reason their weight-loss programme worked this time, rather than any other, was that they were really motivated and committed to their behaviour. The same goes for exercise – every fitness trainer will tell you the one way to succeed with a new exercise programme is by committing yourself to it. Sticking to your diet and exercise programme will be easy – and that guarantees results. Part of the Psychological Solution is, therefore, explaining how you can do just this.

But there's more to the Psychological Solution than just a pep talk. It has been conclusively proven that the way we think and the way our bodies act are intrinsically linked. The reason we are more likely to get sick when we are feeling stressed is because long-term stress actually suppresses the immune system. Conversely, the chemicals produced when we are excited

actually block the cold virus from entering the cells, making it less likely that any bugs will make you sick. Taking this mind-body connection one step further, many diet experts believe that the way we think also changes the way our bodies respond in the presence of food. Awareness of this can help maximize weight loss and help beat cravings and lapses.

And last but not least, as part of the mental makeover, we will tackle the problem of bad body image. It doesn't matter how much weight you lose or how much your cellulite improves, if you have a bad body image you still won't feel happy with yourself. To truly succeed on the plan, you therefore need to turn this around.

CONTENTS

positive thinking

The first step in the Psychological Solution is to get your brain thinking positively about what you can achieve and how you can do it. Many psychologists believe that your brain will strive for what it thinks you want in life, so you need to send out the right messages.

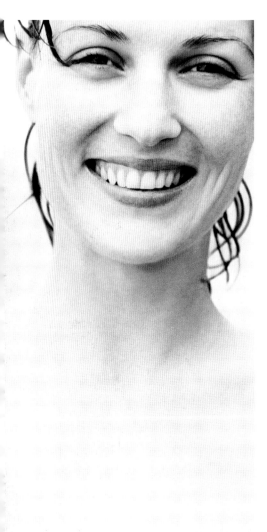

How many times have you looked in the mirror and thought 'I'm too fat', 'I look terrible' or even 'I'm never going to get rid of this cellulite'? Many psychologists believe that if you tell yourself these things, your brain will see them as commands and think 'No, you won't'. They also believe that the brain can't differentiate between positive and negative commands. So if you say to yourself 'I'm not going to fail at this anti-cellulite programme. I will not give up', your brain hears 'I'm GOING to fail and I WILL give up.' It therefore doesn't encourage you to make healthy choices and won't keep you motivated to carry on after the first week.

What is more, negative feelings are stressful, and long-term stress can be a trigger for cellulite, as it increases levels of cortisol (a fat-storage hormone). However, short-term stressors may also cause problems. If you are miserable because you have just broken your diet with a sticky bun, the more you dwell on this, the more stress you are putting yourself under. This causes the release of a whole host of chemicals in the body (including, potentially, cortisol), increasing the chance that the calories in the food you are eating are more likely to turn to fat.

Negative emotions also put our brains out of balance as they are linked to lowered levels of the happy hormone serotonin. One of the fastest ways to get serotonin back into your system is through sweet or starchy food. Perhaps then negative thinking actually triggers food cravings that make it less likely you will stick to your diet plan.

BEATING NEGATIVE THOUGHTS

So how do you get out of the negative thinking trap and into the positive? The simplest way is to use affirmations – every day repeat to yourself what you want to achieve and how you are going to do it. Do this in a positive way: for example, think 'I'm going to fight my cellulite today'. Then you should spell out how; for example, 'I'm going to do my 30-minute walk faster than yesterday. I'm going to eat five portions of fruit and vegetables and I'm going to treat myself to a proper aromatherapy massage.' Tell yourself that three times, or ideally write it down three times, then take the first step to achieve one of those things – grab a banana or make that massage appointment. Remember not to use negative phrasings as they won't inspire your brain to help you.

However, your positive thinking doesn't stop here. You need to affirm what you've achieved at the end of each day. Look at what you wanted to do that day and tick off everything you achieved. If you find something you didn't do, don't beat yourself up; instead look at why and come up with a solution to succeed next time it happens. For example, if you didn't do your walk because it rained all day, could you have walked up and down stairs for 20 minutes in your lunchbreak? The more you come up with solutions, the more successful you'll be.

CULTURAL EFFECTS

Many of us have been trained to think negatively – in many cultures it is more acceptable than thinking well of yourself, which is seen as bragging or unattractive. It has been estimated that by the age of 18, most of us will have been praised 25,000 times (most of these before we were three) – but that we will have received 225,000 negative comments!

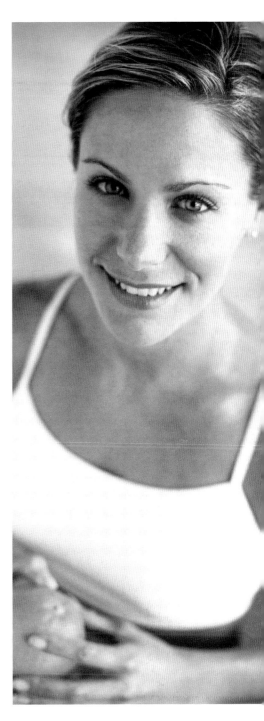

body image

It will be much harder to achieve positive thinking if, every time you look in the mirror, negative feelings creep into your mind because you think you are fat or that you will never succeed because you are a hopeless case. What makes the difference between thinking you're fat (whether you are or not) and knowing you have a few pounds to lose, but not beating yourself up about it, is extremely important when it comes to the success of this plan or any other.

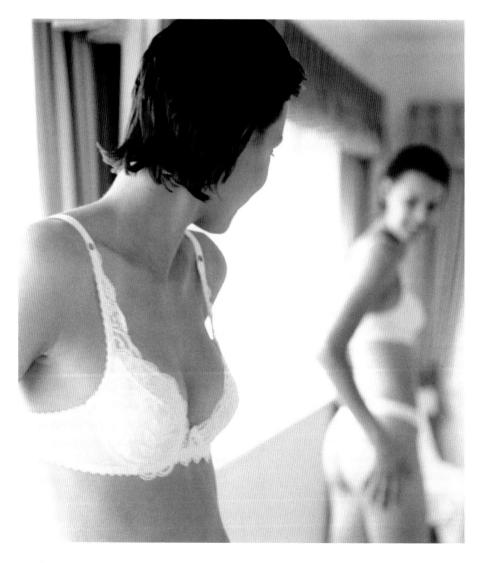

ADAPT YOUR THINKING

1 Think of your trigger factor. Most people with a bad body image didn't develop it themselves. It may have been something said at school or the way your parents nicknamed you 'pudgy' as a child. Look back and try to identify your trigger, then see if it's truly relevant today. Nine times out of ten, it is not.

2 Stop the voice. If a colleague criticized you every time they saw you, you would probably tell them to shut up or stop listening to them. So why do you listen to yourself? Next time you tell yourself that you are fat, start humming, get on the phone or do a few sit-ups to take your mind off your thoughts.

3 Spend two minutes a day standing in front of the mirror looking at yourself – most people who hate their body don't look at it. You will become more neutral about it, and less likely to judge whenever you do catch a glimpse.

4 Get rid of your 'skinny wardrobe'. Sell or give to charity any clothes that don't fit any more. Every time you see them it just reinforces the fact that you are not as thin as you were, and this makes you feel a failure – when in fact you are just normal.

5 Push yourself on the Exercise Solution. Research from the University of South Florida found that just six weeks of exercise dramatically boosted body image – not because the bodies improved, but because the women started to judge their bodies on what they could achieve, not how they looked.

6 Try some flower power. Bach Flower Remedies or Australian Bush Essences take the healing energy of flowers and can help soothe psychological woes. They may work for you.

7 Actually look at other women. Many of us only see other women's bodies in magazines or on TV, and they aren't normal. Look at other women at the gym, on the beach – anywhere – and you'll soon realize that we are supposed to come in sizes both big and small, and that nobody is perfect.

The reason is that if you don't have a healthy body image before you start losing weight, whatever success you have with your cellulite you won't think is good enough. You will still think you've failed, when in fact you've lost 80 per cent of your dimples and look slimmer and trimmer all over. Or while you will be happy with your thighs, you won't be happy with your saggy tummy, which will take the joy out of what you've done. Both of these reactions make it less likely you will maintain the results after the six weeks are up.

CHANGING YOUR IMAGE

Once you are into this success-failure cycle, changing your body can be very hard. Every time you start a diet and fitness programme, you assume (even subconsciously) that it will fail and this makes it harder to start with the positive attitude you need.

Beating a bad body image is therefore vital to success, but it won't be changed overnight. You will probably have felt like this for some time, so it will take a while to adapt your thinking. There are, however, many techniques you can use over the next six weeks to start you on the road. The final part of the Psychological Solution is to carry out one (or more) of the above exercises every day – or whenever you feel you need it.

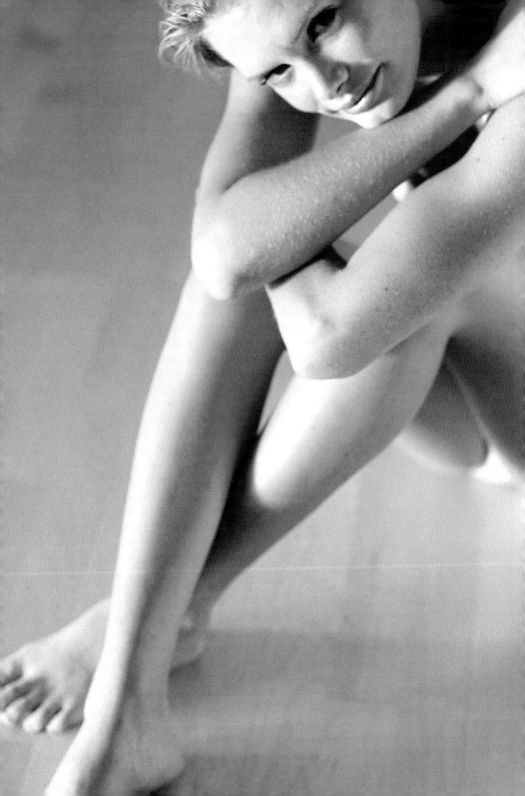

living the
anti-cellulite life

Whether you've been on the plan for six weeks or six months, by the time you have finished the Solutions you should have the results you want. However, if you want your new super-smooth skin to stay that way, you need to know how to maintain your body. As we have seen, there are many elements of modern life that make cellulite almost inevitable, so if you want to break the mould you need to adapt your life to ensure these elements cause less damage.

If you have been following the Solutions for at least six weeks, you will have made a habit of all that good behaviour – your brain is no longer thinking of your new lifestyle as strange, it thinks of it as normal. Therefore, if you go back to a diet of junk food and spend nights on the sofa instead of out for a walk, it will feel just as abnormal as making those positive changes did in the first few weeks of the Solutions. This is great news and you should use it to your advantage, keeping healthy eating and exercise as part of your life. However, this doesn't mean you should still avoid sandwiches for lunch and nights out drinking with the girls every now and again, and can never have a lazy Sunday in bed. Everything in life has a balance and being cellulite-friendly is no exception.

This section will teach you that balance. It will explore what to eat to ensure your diet provides all the benefits of the anti-cellulite plan, but without permanently cutting out bread, sugar or fat. It will look at exactly what exercise you need to keep your new shape – and how to maximize results with the minimum amount of effort. Plus it will explore a whole host of other cellulite-friendly behaviour that will benefit you physically, mentally and cosmetically. In short, it will ensure you are going to love looking in the mirror for quite some time to come.

CONTENTS

what to eat

Adopting a cellulite-friendly diet is one of the most important things you can do to keep the bulges at bay. This takes three steps.

1 WATCH YOUR WEIGHT AND AVOID BINGE-EATING

Maintaining weight can be tricky – you start eating as you used to again and suddenly your weight goes up. Because the Diet Solution doesn't rely on deprivation, you are less likely to want to binge. And if you do want a big night out, have it, as long as you watch what you eat again afterwards.

However, the bad news is that your new thin shape will require fewer calories to maintain it – to truly ensure weight doesn't sneak back on, you have to reassess your calorie needs by working out your metabolic rate once again. Take your weight in pounds (multiply your weight in kilos by 2.22 to find your weight in pounds), and multiply it by 10. Now multiply this figure by the activity factor you used before – see page 25 (remember 1.3 is for totally sedentary workers, 1.7 is for very active workers). The figure you come up with is the number of calories you can eat every day without gaining weight (plus you can add on any extra that you burn during your exercise regime).

Aim to average this intake over seven days, rather than trying to meet it every day. This allows you to have nights out when you don't care what you eat, and then average out the damage over a few days, rather than starving yourself the day afterwards (which often triggers more binge-eating). Finally, weigh yourself once a month and have a weight-gain limit of 1–2 kg (2–4 lb). Should you go over this, cut back on your calorie intake and increase your exercise until you've lost it again.

2 CONTROL FLUID AND PREVENT ITS RETENTION

Remember, it's not just fat that fills the fat 'boxes', fluid can too. While salty foods are no longer banned on your diet plan, you should minimize your intake by choosing low-salt versions of your favourite foods. Again, try not to eat more than 5g (¼oz) of sodium a day. If you do, increase your intake of potassium-heavy foods (like bananas, pears, grapes, leeks and cabbage) as this will help balance out the sodium in your body.

You may also want to start eating wheat again. The good news is that even if you were mildly intolerant to wheat, taking a break from it means your body is going to be less sensitive to it now and you can therefore introduce it back into your eating programme. However, do this gradually – have one meal that includes wheat every other day, then one every day. Work up to two meals that include wheat per day, if you want to.

As you do this, listen to your body: have your bowel movements changed? Are you bloated or gaining weight, despite watching calories? Are you getting headaches, or finding that you are more tired than before? If so, reduce your wheat intake again as you do have a sensitivity and it may be that you need to stick to one meal a day that contains wheat, or even just one a week.

Finally, the easiest way to reduce fluid retention is to stick to those eight glasses of water a day, which will also help distribute nutrients throughout your body and keep your cells shapely and rigid.

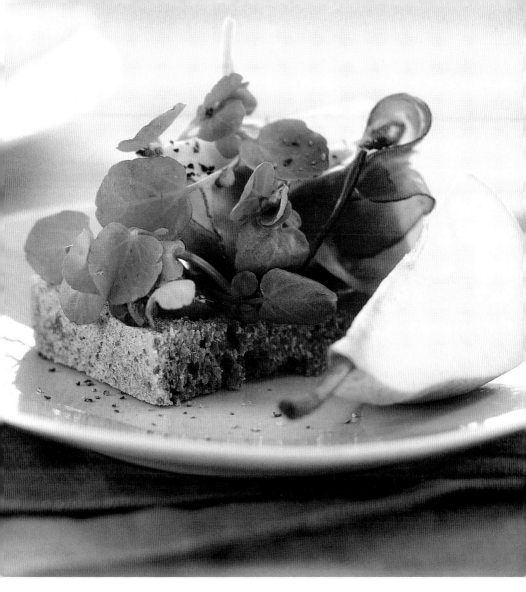

3 FIGHT FREE RADICALS TO REDUCE THE DAMAGE THEY CAUSE

If you have weight and fluid under control, free-radicals are going to be your biggest enemies. Keep supplementing with antioxidant nutrients and stick to the five portions of fruit and vegetables a day, as these have been proven to fight free-radical damage. Try to keep your sugar level low – 40 g (1½ oz) a day is believed to be a safe intake, so read labels carefully. If you have a high-sugar day, increase your intake of broccoli over the next few meals. This contains alpha lipoic acid, which will counteract some of the damage. Fat intake should also be kept low, with no more than 30 per cent of your daily calories coming from fat, and no more than 10 per cent from saturated fat from sources such as butter, fried foods, chocolate and fatty cuts of meat. Again, thinking of this as a weekly limit will make it easier to achieve.

the role of exercise

Hopefully the six weeks you've spent on the Exercise Solution have convinced you how good exercise makes you feel. If so, keep up everything on the programme and the cellulite fighting will continue. You may not feel that way, however.

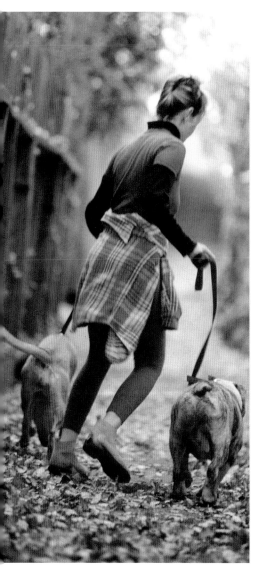

If you weren't quite so sure about all the exercise, at least aim to integrate three 30-minute sessions of activity (such as walking, stair climbing, gardening or dancing) and two toning programmes a week to keep up circulation, muscle mass and calorie burning. Also keep reminding yourself of your correct posture to keep your abductor muscles firm and the lymph flowing freely.

RINGING THE CHANGES

However, whatever level of exercise you decide to do, you'll get better results if you shake your programme up a bit. Our bodies get used to six weeks of the same exercises, so while up until now results will have been steady, you could find they start to slow if you don't change things. Add some different activities to your calorie-burning plans, or if you enjoy what you are doing already, change things about by adding intervals. This means that every 2–3 minutes of your exercise programme, you spend 30–90 seconds working faster or harder.

You will also need to switch things about on the toning plan. To do this, increase the weights you are using or, instead of doing sets of 12 repetitions, get a stopwatch and do as many as you can in 1 minute – and each session try to beat this. Every six weeks, switch things around again (you can go back to your original programme, or start something different again) and remember that the more you challenge your body, the longer it will keep responding.

looking after your skin

In the Beauty and Stimulating Solutions we saw how you can help fight your cellulite by keeping your skin healthy. Now the Solutions have finished, you can drop the weekly massage and hydrotherapy baths, but try to keep up the skin brushing and daily hydration (with or without anti-cellulite cream).

When it comes to the skin's role in preventing more cellulite, the most important thing you can do is step up your sun-care regime. Sun damage causes massive destruction of the collagen and elastin fibres that support the skin and makes the septa shorten and tighten further – making even the limited fat stores you have left more prone to bulging and dimpling. However, 80 per cent of the sun damage we expose our skins to is done by the time we are 18 – it just takes 15–20 years to show up. But this doesn't mean that all is lost; if you start applying sun screen today – and wear it every time you put your skin in the sun – you can actually reverse some of the damage. According to research by Dr Lorraine Kligman at the University of Pennsylvania, when sun screen is applied to the skin every day, it actually begins to grow new collagen within just ten weeks.

USING SUN SCREEN EFFECTIVELY

Research has shown that the majority of us don't use sun screen properly. If you want to live a cellulite-free life, follow these five rules.

1 Choose a sun screen with an SPF (sun protection factor) of at least 15 and make sure it protects against both UVB and UVA rays.

2 Use enough of it or the protection will be reduced. You need a shot glass of sun screen per limb and a teaspoonful for your face.

3 Apply it before you leave home. Sun screens take 20–30 minutes to absorb into the skin.

4 Reapply every 60–90 minutes or after towelling down your body if you are swimming. Waterproof sunscreens will stand up to swimming, but not the action of rubbing yourself dry after your dip.

5 Don't stay out longer than your SPF allows. If you normally burn in 10 minutes, using an SPF 15 means you can stay out for 150 minutes. Reapplying at this point won't protect you any further.

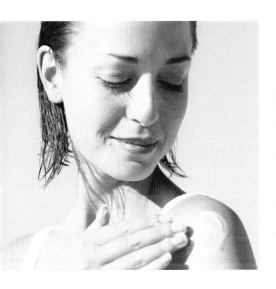

beating bad habits

We've talked about some of the dietary causes of cellulite and how to integrate them safely back into your life after finishing the plan, but here we're going to cover indulgences: things like caffeine, alcohol and cigarettes.

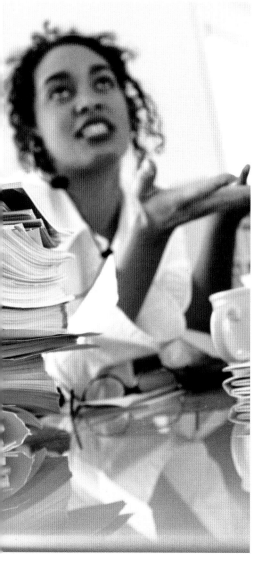

CAFFEINE

While coffee wasn't banned in the Diet Solution, you should have cut down your intake to the recommended 2–3 cups a day. Once your cellulite is beaten, you can increase this to 3–4 cups a day. No health problems have been found from this amount. Don't go over this, though – not only is it bad for your cellulite, but high doses of caffeine have been linked to raised blood pressure and reduced fertility (among other health problems).

ALCOHOL

One alcoholic drink per day was allowed in the Diet Solution, and now you have finished you could even double this and still be within the World Health Organization recommendations for women. But again, keep this as your upper limit – alcohol increases the appetite and could lead you to eat more high-fat, high-sugar foods. Too much alcohol also decreases circulation and may overload the lymph.

CIGARETTES

Up until now we haven't really talked about quitting smoking to fight cellulite – it is probably too daunting a task to add to the programme. However, once you have got all those other healthy habits in place and you are fighting free-radical damage in every other area, perhaps now is the time. There is a very good chance that smoking significantly contributes to cellulite formation, so quitting will therefore help stop its return. The best way to give up smoking for most people is to use nicotine-replacement therapy – success rates on this are double as the lack of withdrawal symptoms (because small doses of nicotine are still provided, usually via patches worn on the skin) makes it easier to break the physical addiction.

Often, however, the habit is harder to break than the nicotine addiction (which actually only lasts 48 hours). You can help yourself by looking at situations when you smoke and have safety tactics in place to counteract the feelings triggering you to light up. These are some good ones to try.

if you smoke when you're stressed

Inhaling oil of lavender is the fastest way to calm your system. Other tactics include drinking camomile tea. See the box on this page for some longer-term approaches to stress.

if you smoke to help you think

Try sniffing peppermint oil or drinking peppermint tea instead. Studies at the University of Cincinnati found this helps people to think more clearly – in fact, those tested scored 28 per cent more highly in accuracy tests than the control group, who didn't sniff any peppermint oil or drink peppermint tea.

if you smoke for something to do

This is quite simple: do something else – doodle, play with computer games, play with stress balls, or anything that keeps your hands busy.

if you smoke to boost energy

Preventing blood-sugar dips that can trigger cravings will help here. Try eating little and often or snack on fruit, which gives your energy a rapid lift without a subsequent fall.

if you smoke out of habit

If you find yourself wanting to smoke when you sit in a particular chair or when you watch a particular television programme, try inhaling some oil of frankincense. This is used to help break ties with the past. The Bach Flower Remedy Honeysuckle has similar effects, and is well worth trying.

CONTROLLING STRESS

Stress can actually cause cellulite by encouraging direct fat storage. Learning to control stress, therefore, can help to control cellulite. Many of us think controlling stress is impossible, but it only takes four steps.

find your triggers

Do you get stressed because you are always waiting for someone else to finish part of a project before you can get your part done? Are you stressed because you can never find your car keys and it makes you late? Think of as many triggers as possible and try to find ways to reduce their effects (an earlier deadline for your colleague, or a key bowl by the front door, maybe).

just say no

Plan your day so you don't take on too much in too short a time, and say no to anything you can't realistically manage.

don't be a worrier

Many of us create stress in our heads by worrying about what might happen. Don't. If something is stressing you, ask yourself what's the worse that could happen – now ask how likely that is. If it is likely, ask how bad it really is. If it is really bad, ask what you can do about it – and take that first step. There aren't many things that really are as bad as we think they could be.

keep your arousal level low

Stress is like a pile of playing cards – you are fine for a while, then something makes everything topple. If you can reduce little stressors (like the noise level in the office or the dripping tap that drives you mad when you work from home), you will reduce the effect that the big stresses can have on you.

index

acknowledgements

Executive Editor: Nicola Hill
Executive Art Editor: Tim Pattinson
Editor: Lisa John
Senior Picture Researcher: Christine Junemann
Production Controller: Nosheen Shan
Designer: Colin Goody
Special Photography: Peter Pugh-Cook
Exercise Consultant: Chrissie Gallagher Mundy

Photography acknowledgements in source order
Alamy /Goodshoot 1, 118
Banana Stock 123
Getty Images /Werner Bokelberg 82 /Robert Bossi 112 /Simon Botttomley 62 /Peter Cade 6-7 /Ken Chernus 14 /Color Day Productions 12 /Chris Craymer 91 /James Darell 2-3 /Davies & Starr 106 /J.P. Fruchet 24 /Michelangelo Gratton 90 /Ray Kachaturian 11 /Rita Maas 30 bottom left /Amy Neunsinger 20 /Photomondo 21 /Stephanie Rausser 122 /Martin Riedl 19 /Marc Romanelli 124 /Spencer Rowell 58 /Steve Taylor 33 bottom left /Julie Toy 92 /Paul Viant 60 /Simon Wilkinson 116 /Roger Wright 114 /Angela Wyant 32 bottom right
Imagestate 109
Octopus Publishing Group Limited 31 bottom left, 38 centre left /Frank Adam 32 top right, 33 bottom right /Stephen Conroy 26, 31 top right, 38 top left /Gareth Sambidge 104, 111 /Jeremy Hopley 10, 22, 33 top right, 121 /Ian Wallace 86, 110 /David Jordan 8, 31 centre left, 36 centre left, 103 top right, 103 bottom right, 103 bottom left /Sandra Lane 32 bottom left, 102 top right /Gary Latham 84 /William Lingwood 30 top right, 30 bottom right, 32 top left, 32 centre left, 33 top left, 40 bottom left /Neil Mersh 30 top left, 46, 51, 55 /Diana Miller 40 centre left, 44 /Sean Myers 33 centre left, 53 bottom right, 103 centre right /Peter Myers 4 /Peter Pugh-Cook 17, 65 left, 65 right, 66 top left, 66 top right, 66 bottom right, 66 bottom left; 67 left, 67 right, 68, 69 left, 69 top right, 69 bottom right, 70 top left, 70 top right, 70 bottom right, 70 bottom left, 70 bottom, 71 top, 71 centre, 72 top left, 72 top right, 72 bottom right, 72 bottom left, 73 top left, 73 top right, 73 bottom, 74, 75 top left, 75 top right, 75 bottom right, 76 top left, 76 top right, 76 bottom right, 76 bottom left, 77 top centre, 77 top right, 77 bottom right, 77 bottom left, 78 top, 78 centre, 78 bottom, 79, 80 top, 80 bottom, 81 top, 81 centre bottom, 81 centre top, 81 bottom, 86 right, 87 top left, 87 top right, 87 bottom right, 87 bottom left, 88, 89 top left, 89 top right, 89 bottom right, 89 bottom left, 94, 95 /William Reavell 5 centre bottom, 28 top left, 28 bottom left, 31 top left, 32 centre right, 36 top left, 40 top left, 42, 48, 52, 96, 102 bottom right, 102 bottom left, 103 top left /Gareth Sambidge 25, 34 /Simon Smith 9, 28 centre right, 29 top left, 29 bottom left /Ian Wallace 29 top right, 29 bottom right, 31 bottom right, 36 bottom left, 54, 57, 102 top left /Philip Webb 38 bottom left, 53 top left /Jacqui Wornell 100 /George Wright 103 centre left
Photodisc 56, 98, 115